THE Men'sHealth®

Belly-Off Program

THE Men'sHealth®
Belly-Off Program

DISCOVER HOW 80,000 GUYS LOST THEIR GUTS . . .
AND HOW YOU CAN, TOO!

Men'sHealth® EDITORS

RODALE

"Belly Busters" illustration © by Zach Trenholm

Photo Credits

Page 14 "Before" and bottom of front cover: Ronald Braun, M.D.; page 14 "After" and color cover photo by Mitch Mandel/Rodale Images; page 20 "Before" and 5th photo on back cover: David Lewis; page 20 "After" and 6th photo on back cover: © by Mike Medby; page 31: Gil Craig; page 41: Geoffrey White; page 47 and 1st photo on front cover: Johnny L. Scott; page 57 "Before": Rey Sifuentes Jr.; page 57 "After": © by James McCoon; page 68 and 1st photo on back cover: Lakin Lankford; page 86 and 3rd photo on front cover: Salvatore Borda; page 98 and 3rd photo on back cover: Michael Stanley; page 109 "Before": Mark Meador; page 109 "After": © by Jeff Adkins; page 128: Mike Brown; page 138 "Before": William Senik; page 138 "After": © by Rodale Inc.; page 148 "Before": Ki Martin; page 148 "After": © by Jason Benkhen; page 162 "Before" and 5th photo on front cover: Jesse Risley; page 162 "After" and 6th photo on front cover: Roark Johnson; page 171: Dennis Vaughn; page 186: Steve Hanzir

Men's Health is a registered trademark of Rodale Inc.

Printed in the United States of America
Rodale Inc. makes every effort to use acid-free ∞, recycled paper ♻.

Text Design by Susan P. Eugster
Cover Design by Charles Beasley

Library of Congress Cataloging-in-Publication Data

The Men's health belly-off program : discover how 80,000 guys lost their guts—and how you can, too! / Men's health editors.
      p.   cm.
Includes index.
ISBN 1-57954-606-4 paperback
1. Men—Health and hygiene.   2. Weight loss.   3. Abdominal exercises.
I. Men's Health (Magazine)
RA777.8 .M463   2002
613'.04234—dc21   2002004339

Distributed to the book trade by St. Martin's Press

2 4 6 8 10 9 7 5 3 1   paperback

Visit us on the Web at www.menshealthbooks.com, or call us toll-free at (800) 848-4735.

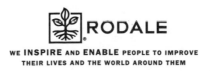

RODALE

WE **INSPIRE** AND **ENABLE** PEOPLE TO IMPROVE
THEIR LIVES AND THE WORLD AROUND THEM

Notice

This book is intended as a reference volume only, not as a medical manual. The information given here is designed to help you make informed decisions about your health. It is not intended as a substitute for any treatment that may have been prescribed by your doctor. If you suspect that you have a medical problem, we urge you to seek competent medical help.

The exercise information in this book is meant to supplement, not replace, proper exercise training. All forms of exercise pose some inherent risks. The editors and publisher advise readers to take full responsibility for their safety and know their limits. Before practicing the exercises in this book, be sure that your equipment is well-maintained, and do not take risks beyond your level of experience, aptitude, training, and fitness. The exercise and dietary programs in this book are not intended as a substitute for any exercise routine or dietary regimen that may have been prescribed by your doctor. As with all exercise and dietary programs, you should get your doctor's approval before beginning.

Mention of specific companies, organizations, or authorities in this book does not necessarily imply endorsement by the publisher, nor does mention of specific companies, organizations, or authorities in the book imply that they endorse the book.

Internet addresses and product information given in this book were accurate at the time this book went to press.

Contents

Part 4: Keeping That Belly Off

Acknowledgments

THIS BOOK RESULTED FROM THE EFFORTS OF MANY TALENTED journalists on the *Men's Health* Books staff. Senior writer Rick Ansorge created early drafts of many of the chapters, with research from Deborah Pedron and Deanna Portz. Rick also interviewed the subjects of our "Belly-Off Success Story" profiles.

Men's Health fitness director Lou Schuler both wrote many of the chapters and served as the book's primary editor. Associate editor Kathryn C. LeSage cleaned up a manuscript written on a tight deadline, while senior development editor Leah Flickinger kept the staff moving forward on multiple projects and contributed some of the writing.

Also deserving a special nod are interior designer Susan P. Eugster and art director and cover designer Charles Beasley.

Office managers Alice Debus and Marianne Moor tackled the daunting task of transcribing tape after tape of Rick's interviews with the "Belly-Off Success Story" guys.

The three big ideas in the Belly-Off Program come from three guys we've interviewed many times over the past few years. We first called Jim Annesi, Ph.D., an exercise psychologist with the YMCA of Metropolitan Atlanta, to find an answer to a perplexing question: Why aren't more men motivated to exercise? You'll probably relate to his impressive insights, which you'll find in chapter 9.

The next person included in this project was trainer and nutritionist Thomas Incledon, R.D., Ph.D., of Plantation, Florida. Tom once said something we've never forgotten: "Weight loss is easy."

Considering that based on the expanding girth of the American population, the opposite would seem to be true, we couldn't wait to hear why he believed something so profoundly counterintuitive. If you can't either, turn to chapter 8.

Following Tom's diet plan and Jim's exercise-adherence plan, you'll find a sample workout routine in chapter 11, courtesy of Craig Ballantyne, C.S.C.S., a consulting strength-and-conditioning coach at McMaster University in Toronto who puts out a fitness-and-sports-training newsletter, e-mailing it to subscribers and posters at his Web site, www.cbathletics.com.

We have to stress that the motivation, diet, and exercise tips in this book aren't the only paths to middle management. They're simply the best we've come across, and the easiest to follow. Each guy who successfully tightens his belt ultimately finds his own way to his goal.

That leads us to the next group of contributors we want to thank here: the men who shared their sometimes painful, sometimes embarrassing, ultimately triumphant stories of taking inches off their waistlines. In particular, we want to express gratitude to Ronald Braun, M.D., who not only offered the tale of dramatic weight loss that appears in chapter 1 but also allowed us to display his before-and-after pictures on the book's cover.

Many of the men profiled achieved their weight loss as members of the *Men's Health* Belly-Off Club, which we started as an offshoot of MensHealth.com in the fall of 2000. The first month, 21,000 guys sign up. By the end of 2001, more than 80,000 were receiving our weekly Belly-Off newsletter. Hundreds of thousands visited the site each month.

Fitness director Lou Schuler deserves credit for conceptualizing an online weight-loss community for men. The people who actually make the site work include director of Internet programming Fred Zahradnik; associate online producer Julie Lubinsky; magazine features editor Tom McGrath; online consumer-marketing manager Claudia Allen; University of Connecticut assistant research professor Jeff Volek, R.D., Ph.D., who answers questions from readers on the Belly-Off message board; and assistant fitness editor Adam Campbell.

Our boss, *Men's Health* vice president and editor-in-chief David Zinczenko, got behind the Belly-Off Club early and often, and championed this book from start to finish.

To all who helped, we hoist a protein shake in your honor.

Introduction

I CAN'T REMEMBER A TIME WHEN I DIDN'T CONSIDER MY FATHER enormously fat. One of my family's favorite stories uses his girth for the punch line. I was 4 years old, and my dad was chasing me through the house, trying to punish me for some infraction or another. (I usually gave my parents multiple choices.) When he finally caught me, I yelled out, "Mom! Get this big gorilla off me!"

Dad laughed so hard he let me go unpunished. To my knowledge, that was the first and last time his weight was cause for laughter.

Many men of his generation had potbellies, and some seemed proud of them, or at least unashamed. To hear Dad tell it, though, his pride of ownership was as large as his belly itself. He wanted us to believe he was fat by ambition and design. "The marines taught me to eat," he would say, implying that my siblings and I were skinny because we hadn't experienced battle. Had we spent years in a military hospital battling dysentery, as he did during World War II, or fighting off communist hordes in Korea, we would have understood that the object of life is to stuff ourselves every chance we get.

I used to look at my dad's obesity two ways: On the one hand, he had grown up in the Depression, served in two wars, and produced seven hungry children—deprivation followed by duty followed by (let's be honest) drudgery. What right did I or anyone else have to judge him for his indulgences? On the other hand,

1

there was something terrifying about the way he indulged, the ferocity with which he ate himself into a stupor every night after work.

No matter how charitable or judgmental I was toward him and the monumental flesh he accumulated, I never imagined that I truly understood him—until I started working on this book.

That's when I saw the connection between cortisol—a stress hormone—and abdominal obesity. Cortisol, as you'll read in chapter 4, not only triggers appetite but also makes sure the extra food you eat gets stored in your midsection, where it can do the most harm.

Dad, the poor bastard, must have been one of the most perfect cortisol-generating machines to ever walk the earth. His anger pulsed to its own beat; no one ever knew when it would erupt into the sort of mayhem that makes psychiatrists see dollar signs.

He didn't die young; he lived to 69, in fact. But his rage ensured that he died alone. He and my mother were long divorced, and only two of his seven children were in contact with him—which explains why he'd been dead for days before anyone realized it.

There's a reason why I'm telling you all this: Most of us in or near the health field (I've been a fitness journalist since 1992) look at weight loss as a mathematical equation no more complicated than balancing a checkbook. Put less in your mouth, put less on your waist. Slow the fork, stop the fat.

As you probably suspect, the issue is far more complex than that. The reasons why people eat too much are hard to quantify. I've already noted my father's unpredictable anger. He was also a chronic gambler, a heavy drinker, and a smoker for most of his adult life. (He was proud when he finally quit smoking, despite the fact that he may have gained as much as 100 pounds in the aftermath.) Though I'm in no way qualified to make psychiatric evaluations, I don't think any weight-loss program would've helped him unless he'd found a way to get all his compulsive and self-destructive behaviors under control.

Perhaps even more insidious than the mental hurdles are the hereditary ones. In fact, as you'll learn in chapter 4, one of the most surprising results of recent research is the way genetics completely obliterates the traditional calorie-counting weight-loss model. You and I can eat the same meal and do the same workout, but I might lose weight and you might gain—or vice versa.

Don't let these obstacles discourage you. Whatever the cause of your weight-control struggle, if you're able to walk into a bookstore and buy this book, I'm confident you can win.

HOW TO USE THIS BOOK

Each guy who buys *The* Men's Health *Belly-Off Program* will use it a little differently. I hope everyone reads the first four chapters, which detail exactly why abdominal fat is different from fat on other parts of your body. I don't mean "different" like "Let's all get along and celebrate diversity." Abdominal fat is different the way that the Khmer Rouge were different from other Cambodians. Left unchecked, it grows ever more evil and rapacious.

I know you'll be tempted to skip past those chapters and go straight to the programs. The diet program, in chapter 8, is unique in that the object is to give you a template for eating right, rather than meal-by-meal specifications. The diet does include very specific sample meals, but not a lifetime's worth. That's why the template is so important: It's a pattern you can follow as long as you want to, without eating the same meals over and over again.

Maybe you'll want to start the book even farther along, flipping back to the exercise chapters, which begin on page 91. There, you'll find an approach to exercise that goes beyond simply expending calories. If you're a guy who has trouble sticking with an exercise program once you've started, you must read chapter 9. The exercise-adherence strategies of Jim Annesi, Ph.D., are the most intriguing I've come across in 10 years of writing fitness articles and books. I think they'll help you better understand your fitness habits, even if you're already a regular weight lifter or runner.

As long as I'm making predictions, my guess is that you're not going to go straight to chapters 14 and 15, which take a close look at weight-loss supplements and last-ditch strategies such as stomach stapling and liposuction. Neither should you ignore them, though, since chapter 14's information on ephedrine may be the most controversial part of this book.

My first instinct as a journalist is to take the easy, government-approved path and tell you, "Don't even consider this stuff." But the ephedrine issue, like everything else involving weight loss, isn't really as black and white as we've been led to believe. The truth is that supplements containing ephedrine and caffeine have been used in weight-loss research and practice for decades, with few side effects. I'm not pushing the stuff, but I can say with confidence that the dangers of ephedrine use as a weight-loss aid have been exaggerated.

Finally, if you picked up this book looking mostly for motivation, you may want to start by reading the profiles of formerly overweight guys that follow each of the 16 chapters. There, you'll find proof that the strategies in this book really work. Some of the guys profiled were fat from childhood but resolved to be lean adults. Some were high school studs who let themselves go before pulling themselves back. These guys lost weight at different ages, in different circumstances, against different odds. What they all have in common is this: They remember the exact moment when they decided they weren't going to be fat anymore. That turning point may have arisen from embarrassment, disgust, a medical emergency, or a personal challenge. Whatever the catalyst, each guy had such a revelation—and each shares his with you in these pages.

Maybe you already had your moment, and it prompted you to pick up this book. Maybe you'll have it while reading these 187 pages. Or maybe another few months or years will pass before you experience it. Whenever that moment occurs, it will prompt you to change not just your body but your entire life. You don't have to take my word for it, though. The former bulk-rate males in this book say it better than I ever could.

Lou Schuler

—LOU SCHULER
FITNESS DIRECTOR
MEN'S HEALTH

Part **1**
The
Scary Part

CHAPTER 1

The Bad News about Your Belly

FRIEND, WE NEED TO TALK ABOUT THAT GUT OF YOURS.

We know you're not proud of it. You may crack jokes about how you're aiming for a gold medal in the splash-diving competition at Athens in 2004. But other than the impressive column of water it helps you spew with each cannonball, you know that belly isn't doing you any good. You don't like looking at it in the mirror, women are turned off by it, children ask if you have a baby in there. You have more trouble sleeping than you used to, your lower back hurts, and exercise makes your knees ache.

But the problem is actually worse than that. Much worse.

Here's a partial list of what happens to you when your waist increases in size.

▶ Your blood pressure rises, putting you at risk for heart disease and stroke.

▶ Your LDL cholesterol—the "bad" form that gums up your arteries—rises.

▶ Your HDL cholesterol—the "good" form that protects against heart disease—falls.

▶ Triglycerides—a type of fat that's a major risk factor for heart disease—rise.

▶ The amount of glucose and insulin in your blood rise, putting you at risk for diabetes.

Accumulating the fat that creates a bigger waistline is effortless and usually fun. To get a beer belly, after all, it helps to drink some beer. But the endgame is brutal: open-heart surgery, blindness, amputation, permanent disability. Premature death could seem like a relief, given the nasty consequences of an unchecked gut.

Belly Busters

▶▶▶ "Last year, on April 1, I attended a family wedding. When I put on my suit, I realized it was extremely tight. I had no option but to suck in my size-40 waist and walk around with my buttocks looking like they were ready to explode out of my pants.

"It was a terrible wake-up call for someone who kept telling himself that despite the fact that he was 5 foot 9 and weighed 225 pounds, he still looked okay. I had truly believed I put it on well.

"The fact that I was constantly tired, suffered from knee problems, and got winded jogging up the stairs hadn't been enough to inspire me. But that incident with the pants totally changed my perspective."◀◀

—RAFFAEL BORELLI
34, LOST 40 POUNDS

Let's get specific: According to the U.S. National Institutes of Health, a waistline bigger than 40 inches for men (35 inches for women) signals significant risk of heart disease and diabetes.

If your waistline is just south of 40, don't breathe a sigh of relief yet. The Canadian Heart Health Surveys, published in 2001, looked at 9,913 people ages 18 to 74 and concluded that the optimal waist size for men is about 35 inches—a little less for younger guys, a little more for older men. Once your unmanaged middle slouches past 35 inches, you're at higher risk of developing two or more of the risk factors for heart disease.

Other studies have found cutoff points between 35 and 40 inches, depending on which risk factors they were studying. But there's a very simple way to sum it all up:

Size-36 pants.

If you can fit comfortably into a pair of pants with a 36-inch waistline, without your belly protruding over your belt, you drastically reduce your risk of developing heart disease and diabetes. It's not a waist size that'll put you in contention for a job as a *Men's Health* cover model, but that's not the goal of this book, either.

Here's what we hope to accomplish in *The* Men's Health *Belly-Off Program.*

▶ Scare the crap out of you by describing the dangers of too much weight in general and too much belly fat in particular. You'll find the ugly details in chapter 3, but here's a preview: About the only major debilitating disease *not* associated with obesity is Alzheimer's.

▶ Look at the most likely reasons why you put on weight in the first place, especially the weight in your midsection. Stress and depression have a lot to do with it, but you're not off the hook for the beer and nachos.

▶ Show you where your diet probably went wrong. You'll never look at "healthy," low-fat food like Nutri-Grain bars the same way again.

▶ Point the way to a healthy diet that will help you lose weight and allow you to keep it off for good. You won't believe how simple this diet is, and you'll be surprised at the strength of the evidence supporting it. You'll wonder why no one told you about it before now.

▶ Map out the three reasons why you may not exercise as much as you want to or should, and show you how to overcome each. Rest assured, the explanation goes deeper than "You're not tough enough." Toughness has nothing to do with it.

▶ Help you decide which form of exercise—strength or endurance—is best for your body type and goals, and present sample programs. This decision is at the heart of the most vitriolic debate in the fitness world today, but research

Belly Busters

▶▶"My weight loss has changed my life. My back pain went away. I now play basketball again and other sports I hadn't realized I missed. [When I play golf,] I walk 18 holes instead of riding a cart. I enjoy feeling like I'm 18 again, and I enjoy being back in the sports world as a participant, not just a spectator."◀◀

—MATTHEW DEISS
31, LOST 100 POUNDS

shows us a simple way to figure out the path to the best possible results.

▶ Examine the "last resort" solutions to your weight problem, including fat-burning supplements (in a stunning upset, we couldn't find much reason to knock ephedrine pills) and liposuction (which makes ephedrine look even better).

▶ Draw up a game plan to help you stick with your diet and exercise goals for life.

THERE'S FAT, AND THEN THERE'S *FAT*

Before we get into the specific problems with—and solutions to—abdominal fat, we need to explain the parameters of the topic. The newest research points toward abdominal obesity—belly fat— as the fastest-growing health risk in America today. So, where possible, we'll focus on belly fat specifically. But much of the research on the dangers of obesity uses a standard called body-mass index, or BMI. This is a simple calculation of a person's weight in relation to his height. A BMI between 25 and 30 indicates that you're overweight; a BMI over 30 signifies obesity. You can check out yours in the chart below.

Body-mass index has one big drawback: It doesn't account for weight distribution. Say you line up three guys who are all 5 foot 10 and 220 pounds. The first guy is a 24-year-old NFL running back with a 33-inch waist. The second guy is a 35-year-old weight lifter with a 36-inch waist. The third guy is a completely sedentary middle-age man with a 40-inch waist. All have a BMI of 31.6, which means that according to U.S. government standards they're all obese.

But they aren't all at equal risk of health problems. The running back, who exercises for several hours a day, is in perfect shape (assuming he doesn't take steroids or massive amounts of painkilling drugs). The weight lifter exercises for several hours a week, and although he carries more fat on his frame than the running back, he isn't going to keel over anytime soon. All that strenuous exertion has made his heart grow bigger and stronger along with his muscles, and he'd be the first guy you'd think of if you needed help carrying a sleeper-sofa upstairs.

The sedentary man, however, is in deep trouble. He may already have

Body Weight (Lb)

Height (In)																	
58	91	96	100	105	110	115	119	124	129	134	138	143	148	153	158	162	167
59	94	99	104	109	114	119	124	128	133	138	143	148	153	158	163	168	173
60	97	102	107	112	118	123	128	133	138	143	148	153	158	163	168	174	179
61	100	106	111	116	122	127	132	137	143	148	153	158	164	169	174	180	185
62	104	109	115	120	126	131	136	142	147	153	158	164	169	175	180	186	191
63	107	113	118	124	130	135	141	146	152	158	163	169	175	180	186	191	197
64	110	116	122	128	134	140	145	151	157	163	169	174	180	186	192	197	204
65	114	120	126	132	138	144	150	156	162	168	174	180	186	192	198	204	210
66	118	124	130	136	142	148	155	161	167	173	179	186	192	198	204	210	216
67	121	127	134	140	146	153	159	166	172	178	185	191	198	204	211	217	223
68	125	131	138	144	151	158	164	171	177	184	190	197	203	210	216	223	230
69	128	135	142	149	155	162	169	176	182	189	196	203	209	216	223	230	236
70	132	139	146	153	160	167	174	181	188	195	202	209	216	222	229	236	243
71	136	143	150	157	165	172	179	186	193	200	208	215	222	229	236	243	250
72	140	147	154	162	169	177	184	191	199	206	213	221	228	235	242	250	258
73	144	151	159	166	174	182	189	197	204	212	219	227	235	242	250	257	265
74	148	155	163	171	179	186	194	202	210	218	225	233	241	249	256	264	272
75	152	160	168	176	184	192	200	208	216	224	232	240	248	256	264	272	279
76	156	164	172	180	189	197	205	213	221	230	238	246	254	263	271	279	287
BMI	19	20	21	22	23	24	25	26	27	28	29	30	31	32	33	34	35

Syndrome X, a deadly stew of high blood pressure, high triglycerides, low HDL cholesterol, and high blood sugar. From Syndrome X, it's a short hop to diabetes type 2, heart disease, or both.

So any measure that puts a professional athlete, a dedicated exerciser, and a completely sedentary man in the same category is too crude to be useful to an entire population—it can't distinguish between muscle and fat, or between active overweight people and inactive ones. That's why researchers began using waist size to determine health risks.

Waist size is more useful than BMI for two important reasons.

1. Fat that pushes your waist out in front is most likely visceral fat, meaning it's probably behind your abdominal muscles and surrounding your internal organs. This is the most dangerous kind of fat you can have on your body. A study at the University of Alabama–Birmingham published in 1997 in *Medicine and Science in Sports and Exercise* sums it up: The researchers took 137 men and used seven different measurements to determine their risks of cardiovascular disease. They found that the amount of visceral fat the men carried was the single best sign of multiple heart-disease risks.

2. Waist size can be an indicator of how much exercise you get. Exercise attacks visceral fat, so the more visceral abdominal fat you have, the more likely it is that you don't get a healthy amount of exercise.

Belly Busters

▶▶"Toward the end of college and for a couple of years after that, I worked several jobs at once, including an overnight radio gig that disrupted my sleep cycle. I ate when I could and whatever was convenient. If that meant a half-gallon of whole milk and a box of mini powdered doughnuts while I worked, I figured, 'So?'

"Around 1994, I went for a physical exam after several years of not having one. I found out my real weight: 247. My cholesterol and blood pressure were embarrassing. I also smoked. Finally, in 1997, I asked myself, 'What would life be like if I weren't embarrassed to take off my shirt to go swimming? What would it be like to enter a room and not feel self-conscious?' I had hated the idea of moving up to size-40 pants.

"I began walking every night. I also stopped bringing foods like cheese, bacon, and whole milk into my apartment. Soon some pounds came off.

"I'm now at 190 pounds with a 34-inch waist. My cholesterol and blood pressure are fine. I'm sorry I didn't make these changes earlier."◀◀

—STEVEN KLAPOW
32, LOST 57 POUNDS

Waist size still isn't a perfect measure of health risk, since fat around your waistline could include less-dangerous subcutaneous fat that is right beneath your skin and doesn't affect your organs. (Subcutaneous waist fat is better known as love handles.) So researchers also use waist-hip ratio to assess health risks. If a guy's hip circumference is bigger than his waist size, he's generally in better shape than a guy whose waist

Belly Busters

▶▶ "The summer after my first year of teaching high school, I weighed in at 355 pounds. I am 6 foot 3 and was always told, 'You're just a big guy.' Two weeks before the summer ended, I visited my best friend in Nashville. We were just chilling out at the pool one day, when an older gentleman came by. He began talking about training for a marathon. The thought hit me, 'I hope I am in that kind of shape when I get to his age.' Then I realized that at the rate I was going, I would never even live to his age.

"That day, a lot of things crossed my mind, and I decided I was going to lose the weight and keep it off. A year and a half later, I'm down to 220. I went from a 56-inch chest to a 46, and from a 48-inch waist to a 36."◀◀

—SCOTT THORNE
30, LOST 125 POUNDS

is bigger than his hips. A 2001 study published in the *American Journal of Clinical Nutrition* found that a bigger hip circumference in men correlates to less visceral fat and more muscle mass.

The classic example of a guy with a threatening waist-hip ratio is the doofus who brags that he's still wearing the same size-32 Levi's he wore in high school. He's telling the truth, although he doesn't mention that the fly of those Levi's now resides in permanent darkness beneath his overhanging belly. While his hips and every other part of his body are the same size they were back in his glory days (or perhaps are even smaller, due to muscle loss), he has gotten bigger in the most dangerous place.

All that said, when you look at the general population, you won't find a huge statistical difference between BMI, waist size, and waist-hip ratio as predictors of health risks. Few of us are like the handful of NFL running backs and dedicated weight lifters who carry a lot of weight that isn't fat.

THE GIRTH OF A NATION

In 1960, 45 percent of American adults were over their ideal weight: 31.6 percent were overweight, and an additional 13.4 percent were obese. In 1999, according to the U.S. surgeon general's report, 61 percent of American adults were overweight, with 27 percent classified as obese.

In other words, our national fatness level has almost doubled in the span of 4 decades, with most of the increase occurring during the 1990s.

Most disturbing? The youngest adults are gaining weight the fastest. Check out these numbers from a 2001 study in the *Journal of the American Medical Association*.

Age Group	Rate of Obesity Increase 1991–98
18–29	69.9%
30–39	49.5%
40–49	34.3%
50–59	47.9%

Here's the price we all pay for this unprecedented population widening.

▶ Today, obesity kills an estimated 300,000 Americans each year.

▶ Obese people have a 50 to 100 percent higher overall risk of premature death than people of normal weight. Cardiovascular diseases cause most of the increased risk. And the longer you stay obese, the closer you get to the higher number.

▶ Even though driving while fat is not a crime, obesity is as likely to kill you as heavy drinking, according to a national study of 9,585 adults. It's also associated with at least as much morbidity as cigarette smoking and poverty.

▶ Obesity is even more likely than heavy drinking, cigarette smoking, or impoverishment to cause serious disease. Obese adults have almost two times as many chronic illnesses as people of normal weight.

▶ Caring for obesity-related disease accounts for 9.4 percent of U.S. healthcare expenditures. Direct and indirect costs of obesity and overweight are nearly $100 billion a year, including $4 billion a year in lost productivity (meaning the value of wages lost by people who can't work because they are sick or disabled, as well as the value of future earnings lost because of premature death). By contrast, cigarette smoking indirectly costs the nation about $48 billion a year.

▶ In one study, 28 percent of teachers said that becoming obese is "the worst thing that can happen to a person" and 24 percent of nurses said they are "repulsed" by obese people. These statements suggest widespread prejudice against fat people, even as the population gets more widespread.

▶ A Michigan State University study found that overweight and obese people

Belly Busters

▶▶ "Three weeks into my marriage, after having these hot buffalo wings for dinner, something didn't seem right. My heart was beating irregularly and fast. I was hesitant to say something to my wife, but it kept getting worse.

"The next minute I knew, I was in the hospital overnight with an irregular heartbeat that was 165 beats per minute. It scared me to death. All I could think about was getting a second chance.

"I did a 360 with my lifestyle. I never used to do cardio workouts, only strength training. I bought a treadmill that I use in the mornings, three times a week. I cut back on heavy weights by doing more repetitions on lower weights. I also got a dog to force me to take daily walks.

"My wife is from Switzerland, and the house is full of cheese, chocolate, and Swiss mayo. I stopped eating that stuff and started to eat more greens. More important, I stopped eating 2 hours before bed. I used to put gravy on my fries, rice, or potatoes. I removed that because my cholesterol was high. Broccoli is now my best friend, and water is my mistress."◀◀

—EARL HUNTER
33, LOST 18 POUNDS

almost never show up on TV. When big guys make it onto the airwaves, they're rarely depicted having a good time with friends ("Hello, *Newman*") or getting it on with romantic partners. They are, however, more likely to be shown eating than are normal and underweight male characters.

Scared? Bewildered? Pissed off? Good. Now let's meet your belly fat, up close and visceral.

The Doctor Is Thin

LIFE IN THE FAT LANE

During his roly-poly college years, Ronald Braun loved playing the jovial fat guy. One of his favorite antics was to outsmart the workers who ran the "Guess Your Weight" game at an area amusement park.

"Their scales only went to 300 pounds, so it was impossible for them to measure my weight," he says. "My big joke was to visit the park and win free gifts."

Sometimes, however, the joke was on him.

He once climbed aboard an amusement ride that seated 10 people in each row. A safety gate was supposed to secure all 10 snugly in place. "I was the only person it didn't fit, so I had to get out of the ride," says Dr. Braun.

Dr. Braun's struggle with his weight began in junior high school. Both his parents worked long hours to make ends meet, so he ate many of his meals at fast-food restaurants.

Through high school, Dr.

Braun's weight held steady at about 270 pounds, partly because he played sports.

After graduating, however, Dr. Braun enrolled in an accelerated medical-school program that crammed undergraduate work and med school into 6 years. Squeezed for time, he subsisted on fast-food hamburgers, french fries, pizza, and soft drinks.

"I drank almost 4 liters of Pepsi or Coke a day," he says. "That was almost 2,500 calories in soft drinks alone."

Since he never exercised, it was only a matter of time before he became as supersize as his fast-food meals. Three years into the program, he weighed 330 pounds and had a 44-inch waist.

His blood pressure became dangerously high. At night, he often awoke suddenly to catch his breath. "Although I was never diagnosed, I believe I had sleep apnea," he says.

THE TURNING POINT

In medical school, Dr. Braun became friends with another overweight student.

"One day he said, 'I'm going to eat better,'" Dr. Braun recalls. "He didn't do anything crazy or bizarre, and he went from 260 pounds to 180 pounds in 7 or 8 months."

Dr. Braun was awestruck. So were the other medical students—especially the women, who took special note of his friend's spud-to-stud transformation.

Dr. Braun knew his girth had prevented him from enjoying

Name: RONALD BRAUN, M.D.
Date of Birth: December 1970
Residence: Ft. Lauderdale
Occupation: Anesthesiologist
Height: 6 foot 3

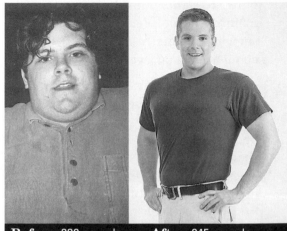

Before: 330 pounds   **After:** 245 pounds

everything life has to offer. But until his friend's transformation, it hadn't occurred to him that his size wasn't a life sentence.

"He was an amazing inspiration. I thought, 'If he can do it, I can do it.'"

THE PLAN OF ATTACK

Dr. Braun's first step was to switch from regular soda to diet and stop eating fried foods. "I lost about 25 pounds, but then I plateaued," he says.

That prompted him to start counting calories and grams of fat, to stop eating hamburgers and steaks, and to start eating more chicken and fish. He achieved dramatic results: Within 9 months, he was down to 215 pounds and a 34-inch waist.

After graduating from medical school, he began his residency at the prestigious Johns Hopkins University Hospital in Baltimore, and started using the weight machines in the hospital's cardiac-rehab unit.

Despite working up to 120 hours a week, Dr. Braun hit the weights for an hour to an hour-and-a-half three times a week. Whenever he could spare a few extra minutes, he added some cardiovascular exercise.

Proud of his transformation from a 330-pound hulk to 245-pound hunk with a 36-inch waist, he resolved to continue exercising even if his bosses made him work 200-hour weeks.

LIFE IN THE FIT LANE

Looking back, Dr. Braun marvels at how a commitment to diet and exercise has changed his life. As his blood pressure nose-dived to normal, his self-esteem and social status soared.

"I felt so much better and had so much more energy," he says.

At his 10-year high school reunion, Dr. Braun had to carry an old photograph to help his classmates remember him.

Five years after losing weight, Dr. Braun stays true to his twin callings: medicine and fitness.

Now an anesthesiologist working up to 80 hours a week at a Ft. Lauderdale hospital, he still shuns fast food, soda, and snacks, and eats three low-fat meals a day. "I strive for about 3,000 calories and less than 30 grams of fat a day," he says.

He still lifts weights three or four times a week, and also works out on an exercise bike

and stairclimber. He recently took up jogging.

In the hospital's operating room, Dr. Braun works alongside a doctor who performs stomach-stapling surgery. "Every day, I see obese patients whose only option is to have their stomachs stapled," he says.

Dr. Braun knows that, but for the grace of God—and a lot of discipline and hard work—he, too, could have ended up with a stapled stomach that can accommodate only one chicken wing for dinner.

"It makes me proud that I did it the way I did," he says. "I will never, ever be that size again. Now I'm somebody different."

HIS TIPS

Like many doctors, Dr. Braun constantly hears people complain that they don't have time to exercise. If he wanted to get up on his high horse, he could tell them that *he* finds time to exercise, despite working 70 to 80 hours per week.

"So many people think it's an extracurricular thing," he says. "Exercise is not optional. It's something that has to be done as part of the routine maintenance of our bodies."

The Enemy Within

IF YOU'RE AN AVERAGE GUY, YOU HAVE ABOUT 30 BILLION FAT CELLS, each of them resembling a tiny water balloon filled with greasy substances called lipids.

Like a water balloon, a fat cell has the ability to expand. It can grow up to 1,000 times its original size.

Unlike a water balloon, however, it doesn't burst. Once it reaches a certain size, it subdivides, leaving you with two fat cells instead of one. Unfortunately, the process doesn't work in reverse; once you have a fat cell, you're stuck with it for life. So if you double the number of fat cells in your body, you double the difficulty you'll have losing the lipids inside them.

It's easy to look down at that lipid retirement community between your nipples and navel and figure you have all the time in the world to get rid of its deadbeat tenants. Unfortunately, abdominal fat doesn't just sit there waiting for an eviction notice. It's metabolically active tissue that functions like a separate organ, releasing many different substances that can either help you or harm you.

BAD FAT

The notion that abdominal obesity is the most dangerous kind isn't new. Back in the 1940s, French physician Jean Vague observed that some obese patients had normal blood chemistry and blood pressure, while some moderately overweight patients showed serious abnormalities that predisposed them to heart disease or diabetes.

Almost always, the moderately overweight patients carried their fat around their middles. And, almost always, they were men.

Since men are genetically programmed to accumulate visceral abdominal fat, we become what is commonly known as *apple-shaped*. To better describe this high-risk form of obesity, Dr. Vague coined the term *android* (male-type) obesity. Android is a good way to characterize your belly fat. While the word *apple* implies that something healthy is going on down there, anyone with a casual knowledge of science fiction knows an android can take on a life of its own once you've created it.

A few unfortunate women are also apple-shaped, which raises their heart-disease risk as high as a man's, especially if they gain weight in their midsections before menopause. Most women, however, are genetically programmed to gain weight in their thighs and buttocks. Dr. Vague coined the term *gynoid* to describe this type of fat. Since this isn't the sort of word you want to use in mixed company (unless you want to feel a sharp elbow in your

Belly Busters

▶▶ "On January 11, 1998—yes, I remember the exact date—I put on a pair of size-42 pants I had just gotten a couple of weeks before and found them too tight. Ugh! I was pushing 250 pounds at a recent physical exam. (I am 6 foot 1). I had a desk job at a local bank and got absolutely no exercise, ever. I had 'banker's butt' at age 28. I wasn't getting any younger. Something had to change, and I had to do it. No one could do this for me but me.

"Losing the weight and getting into shape is far and away the greatest achievement of my life. I still have a desk job, but now that I exercise regularly, I don't worry about 'banker's butt' anymore. I am living proof that you can do it if you only get off the couch and try.

"Last week, I gave away some of my old suits to the rummage sale at my aunt's church. I tried one of them on and cracked up at the sight of myself in my 'fat clothes.' There was room for me and a friend." ◀◀

—MARK OHLINGER
31, LOST 60 POUNDS

androids), we usually use the more common term *pear-shaped* to describe less harmful, slow-growing, below-the-waist fat.

Multiple studies following Dr. Vague's pioneering work have shown that abdominal fat is more than nature's way of telling you that you'll never become a soap opera star, news anchor, rock legend, or *Men's Health* cover model. It's a sign that your body chemistry is seriously out of whack.

Abdominal fat cells contain high levels of lipoprotein lipase, an enzyme that makes them soak up excess calories and expand to their outer limits. So you may not be exaggerating when you complain that every doughnut you eat goes straight to your gut. You may simply be stating a scientific fact.

Since abdominal fat literally resides within striking distance of your heart, liver, and other vital organs, it's in a position to commit much more mayhem than other fat. It does its dirty work by secreting excessive amounts of substances that increase your risk of disease. These include:

Free fatty acids. Released directly to the liver, free fatty acids impair your ability to break down the hormone insulin, so you have too much of it circulating in your system. Over time, your body develops insulin resistance, a condition that often leads to diabetes. Free fatty acids also prompt the liver to overproduce triglycerides, blood fats that increase your risk of heart disease.

Cortisone. High levels of this hormone are associated with diabetes and high blood pressure.

PAI-1. This molecule fat releases is a blood-clotting agent that increases your risk of heart attacks and strokes.

CRP. This protein promotes inflammation that damages blood vessels, making them more susceptible to artery-clogging plaque.

Tumor necrosis factor (TNF) alpha. In lean people, this helps regulate the metabolic and immune systems. In obese people, however, excessive amounts of TNF alpha can result in insulin resistance and increased fat storage.

Aromatase. As body weight increases, this enzyme creates a vicious cycle in which you gain more and more weight around your middle.

By now, it should be obvious that android fat is a chemical-weapons factory. Even more ominously, it's a chemical-weapons factory that, like a misprogrammed robot, proceeds with its own agenda. Here's some more scary proof.

In 2001, Johns Hopkins University School of Medicine researchers grew fat cells and nerve cells in a container, separated by a thin membrane. They found that the fat cells signaled the nerve cells to increase production of a chemical called neuropeptide Y, or NPY. NPY signals your brain to (1) stop burning fat, and (2) stimulate your appetite. Obviously, both of these effects make you fatter.

You can guess which kind of fat contains the greatest number of NPY-

Belly Busters

▶▶ "I got my jawline back. I look better, feel better. And, yes, I can once again see my tree of life, which had been shaded by my gut. Oh yeah, skinny sex is much better than fat sex, and slimming down creates much more opportunity." ◀◀

—JAMES GORDON
44, LOST 60 POUNDS

producing nerve cells: the Big A—also known as abdominal fat, android fat, and apple fat.

This study suggests that your gut may actually possess a primitive form of intelligence. Your fat cells may be so smart that they know how to protect themselves and increase their numbers.

And you thought *Invasion of the Body Snatchers* was scary.

NOT-SO-BAD FAT

Once you accept that visceral abdominal fat is different from the other fat on your body, a logical question arises: Is the other fat bad for you? In other words, if you lost most of your visceral fat but still had large quantities of subcutaneous fat jiggling around on your love handles and jowls, would you be any less healthy than a guy with no jiggles?

Maybe, but maybe not.

The University of Alabama–Birmingham study mentioned in chapter 1 included a startling discovery: Fat on your legs is a sign of *reduced* heart-disease risk in both men and women. Specifically, people with larger thighs have lower triglycerides and fewer of the lowest-density cholesterol molecules, the ones that form artery-clogging plaque.

Another clue that subcutaneous fat isn't all that dangerous comes from sumo wrestlers. When Japanese researchers studied 15 of them, they found that these obviously obese athletes were in surprisingly good shape. Tests revealed that they had relatively little visceral fat, and blood screenings

 Belly Busters

▶▶"Our fire department has been taking on a few new members in the past year. These guys are young and in shape. [They] look up to us for guidance and training, but I wondered what they really saw. A bunch of old guys who were out of shape and would probably have a heart attack on the fire ground?

"I started taking a closer look at myself. I had a 35-inch waist. I looked through my closet and brought out a pile of clothes I used to wear and tried them on. I was shocked at how I looked. I was currently wearing only large sweatshirts, which hid everything quite well. Wearing shorts or T-shirts was out of the question.

"So I thought about exercising and changing my eating habits. I'd tried this before and was unsuccessful. But I decided to try again.

"This time it was different. It worked."◀◀

—JEFF SOVERAN
39, LOST 42 POUNDS

showed that they had low cholesterol and normal levels of triglycerides and blood sugar.

Bear in mind that all of this doesn't necessarily mean you should learn to accept and love your love handles. The UAB researchers also found that subcutaneous abdominal fat does have some correlation to heart-disease risk, though the link is not as strong as that between visceral fat and cardiovascular problems.

That Dam Gut

LIFE IN THE FAT LANE

As a young adult, David Lewis had a knack for keeping his chubbiness in check. He joined a gym, watched what he ate, and kept his weight steady at 165 to 170 pounds.

Then, in 1996, he took a job that required him to work 14- to 16-hour days.

"I very gradually stopped going to the gym and eating right," he says. "I'd come home, eat dinner, and go right to sleep."

In 1998, Lewis married his longtime girlfriend, Jeannie.

"Jeannie and I share the household responsibilities, and I found out I was pretty good in the kitchen," he says. "It wasn't a question of watching the calorie or fat intake. If it looked good and tasted good, I cooked it and we ate it."

It didn't take long for this high-pressure, activity-free, pasta-rich lifestyle to take its toll on his waistline. Within 3 years, his weight had ballooned to 240 pounds, and he was wearing size-44 pants.

"I realized what was happening," he says. "I just didn't take any action."

Unlike many middle-age guys, Lewis could console himself with the fact that his problems were primarily cosmetic. "I wasn't having any kind of medical problems," he says.

Still, he had a nagging suspicion that all was not well.

"I wasn't feeling the way I should feel," he says. "I was feeling tired. I didn't have the energy I needed."

THE TURNING POINT

By 2001, Lewis was working a saner schedule: 6:30 A.M. until 4:00 P.M. But he hadn't yet straightened out his eating and exercise habits. He experienced what he calls his *click moment* that July, after he and Jeannie returned from a vacation in Las Vegas.

"I wasn't feeling sick," he says. "But my energy levels were really low."

At first, he thought it was the summer heat. Then he saw some digital photos from his recent vacation on his home computer. As he gazed at a photo of himself standing on the edge of Hoover Dam, he felt as *wide* as Hoover Dam.

Fortunately, his initial self-disgust was overwhelmed quickly by self-resolve: "I just said to myself, 'Hey, that's it. I've got to fix it.'"

The next day, he told Jeannie he was joining a gym and asked if she wanted to join, too.

Without hesitating, she said, "Yeah, let's go."

Name: DAVID LEWIS
Date of Birth: December 1955
Residence: Yorba Linda, California
Occupation: Service/training manager
Height: 5 foot 9

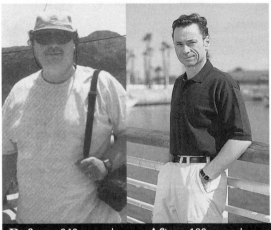

Before: 240 pounds   **After:** 160 pounds

THE PLAN OF ATTACK

Lewis set an ambitious goal: to be 180 pounds lighter by January 1, 2002.

"I know what I had to do," he says. "I knew I had to fix my eating habits, and I knew I had to get out and exercise."

Lewis placed himself on a 1,500-calorie diet, eating five or six small meals a day. He switched from bread, pasta, and other starches to fresh fruits, vegetables, and other "clean carbs." He gave up red meat in favor of turkey, chicken, and fish. He allowed himself no alcoholic beverages, and drank 100 to 120 ounces of water a day to control his appetite.

At the gym, Lewis started with a stationary bicycle. "At first, I could only do 15 minutes before I gave out," he says. He gradually increased his stamina, to 30 minutes after 2 weeks and 45 minutes after 6 weeks. Soon, he felt strong enough to step onto a stairclimber and tackle strength training.

"The first 2 weeks, I dropped over 10 pounds," says Lewis. "Although a lot of it was water loss, it was pretty encouraging to see those first pounds come off."

Since Lewis was working out 7 days a week, he kept losing weight at a steady clip and never hit a plateau. "My routine was pretty intense, and I stuck with it," he says. "I didn't take any cheat days. The more I succeeded, the more motivation I had to keep going."

Lewis tracked his progress on the same computer that had given him such a rude shock. He achieved his goal of shedding 180 pounds months ahead of schedule. By December 2001, he weighed 160 pounds and wore size-32 pants.

LIFE IN THE FIT LANE

Because of his determination, the onetime O-shaped Lewis became the proud owner of a V-shaped physique.

"I feel better than I have in 10 years," he says. "My energy levels are up, I require less sleep, and I look great. I'm in better shape now than when I graduated from college."

He has given away all his old clothes and has no intention of ever needing them back.

After he stabilized at 160 pounds, Lewis began gradually increasing the amount of food he ate. Not wanting to live like a monk, he also allowed himself an occasional beer or margarita.

But he still works out hard: up to 2 hours a session, 6 days a week.

"I'm very comfortable with the 160, so I don't plan on dropping any more weight," he says. "Now my objective is to build some lean muscle."

HIS TIPS

BE CREATIVE. "If you want it bad enough, you'll figure out a way to make it happen."

MAKE EXERCISE A HABIT. "The first thing I do after I get home from work is drop off my stuff and head to the gym."

MIX UP YOUR ROUTINE. "If something's not working for you, don't be afraid to make an adjustment."

ENLIST YOUR SPOUSE. "Although Jeannie wasn't as strict as I was, she dropped 20 to 25 pounds. She's been a great support for me, and she looks fabulous."

KEEP YOUR FAT PHOTOS. "I have two of them on my refrigerator door. As painful as they are for me to look it, they remind me that I don't want to go back to where I was."

Corpulence
Attacks!

AS WE BEGAN RESEARCHING THIS BOOK, WE COMPILED A LIST OF ALL the diseases associated with abdominal obesity. We ended up with a total of 39 conditions, from acanthosis nigricans to urinary stress incontinence. (See page 24 for the complete list—and to find out what the hell *acanthosis nigricans* is.)

Let's take a look at the most common ways belly fat can ruin your health.

DIABETES TYPE 2

Researchers estimate that about 16 million Americans have diabetes, with at least a third of those cases undiagnosed and untreated. The disease is the seventh-leading cause of death in America. The overwhelming majority of cases—90 to 95 percent—are diabetes type 2 (formerly known as adult-onset diabetes), the kind most closely linked to obesity. (People with diabetes type 1 are usually diagnosed as children. They have a congenital inability to produce insulin, the hormone that shuttles blood sugar into muscle, fat, and other cells.)

Diabetes type 2 usually starts with insulin resistance. Here's how it works: After you eat a meal, your body has more blood sugar, or glucose, than it can use for energy at that moment. So it releases insulin to transport the excess glucose into your muscles and other places where it can be stored for future use.

If your body's tissues become resistant to insulin, or less sensitive to its actions, your glucose has no place to go. Some gets turned into fat, but the rest can become toxic and damage blood vessels.

At first, your pancreas produces more insulin to get the surplus glucose out of your bloodstream. When it stops producing this extra insulin, you have diabetes. And then you could feel the effects in any number of ways. You might suffer damage to your nerves (which can lead to amputations), retinas (which can lead to blindness), bones, or kidneys. About 75 percent of patients with diabetes type 2 die from arteriosclerosis, or hardening and thickening of the arteries.

A quick tip-off that you have diabetes: You get sleepy right after a meal. Other signs include frequent urination and increased thirst (your body dehydrates itself as it desperately tries to get rid of the glucose), nausea, and blurred vision. Two others: Your wife will notice that your breath smells like nail polish remover, and your doctor will notice that your blood pressure is elevated.

This miserable disease, which you shouldn't wish on your worst enemy, is almost entirely self-inflicted. Being overweight and inactive are important nongenetic risk factors. For every

Belly Busters

▶▶"At age 40, I weighed 250 pounds and had chronic lower-back pain, high blood pressure, sleep apnea, and borderline diabetes. I'd had enough of being tired and sluggish, and watching my health deteriorate. I could not even walk a half-mile without doubling over from back soreness and strain. My doctor suggested I lose weight. Since then, I have lost 41 pounds. I no longer have high blood pressure, back pain, or abnormal blood sugar, and my doctor is going to reassess my sleep apnea so that I can sleep without a mask on my face."◀◀

—DAVID RICHARDSON
42

pound you gain, your diabetes risk increases about 2 percent. So if you've put on 50 pounds since college, you're twice as likely to get diabetes as your college roommate who stayed at his fighting weight.

As you've probably guessed, carrying that extra weight in your abdomen puts you at particular risk. A Dutch study found that men whose waist circumferences were larger than 40 inches were nearly eight times as likely to have diabetes as men whose waists measured less than 37 inches. Another study found that among Hispanics and African-Americans with family histories of diabetes, belly fat is an even greater risk factor for insulin resistance than age, gender, or overall weight.

Researchers aren't sure why excess fat causes insulin resistance. Some believe that fat cells may produce a substance—a hormone they've dubbed *resistin*—that blocks the passage of insulin into muscles and other cells. Resistin has shown up in animal studies, but researchers aren't sure whether human fat cells produce it.

CARDIOVASCULAR DISEASE

Before we get into the links between cardiovascular disease and obesity, we should define a few terms so we don't get bogged down in them. Most of the conditions we'll be describing have more than one name. We'll use the terms *cardiovascular disease* and *heart disease* interchangeably to describe a class of disorders that affect the heart or its blood vessels. About 61 million Americans are affected by such conditions, which include arteriosclerosis, heart attack, stroke, and high blood pressure, and the annual death toll is about one million.

Big Concerns: The Complete List

- Acanthosis nigricans (dark, thick, velvety skin in body folds and creases)
- Arthritis
- Cancer
- Cardiovascular disease
- Carpal tunnel syndrome
- Cataracts
- Chronic hypoxia and hypercapnia (respectively, decreased oxygen and increased carbon dioxide in tissue)
- Chronic pain
- Chronic venous insufficiency (blood vessels do not channel bloodflow properly and fail to efficiently return blood to the heart)
- Daytime sleepiness
- Deep venous thrombosis (blood clotting in a deep vein)
- Diabetes type 2

- Elephantiasis
- Endocrine, or hormonal, abnormalities (reduced testosterone levels, breast cancer in men, hypertension, impotence, male infertility, respiratory distress syndrome, stress-related diseases)
- Gallbladder disease
- Gastroesophageal reflux
- Gout
- Gum disease
- Heat injury, disorders, and intolerance
- Heel spurs
- Hernias
- Hypertension
- Impaired immune response
- Impaired respiratory function
- Infections following wounds

- Kidney disease
- Liver disease
- Lower-back pain
- Lower-extremity edema
- Pancreatitis
- Panniculitis (inflammation in the fatty layer under the skin on the front of the abdomen)
- Pseudotumor cerebri, or benign intracranial hypertension (increased pressure within the skull)
- Skin problems (due to trapped secretions and friction between skin folds)
- Sleep apnea
- Stroke
- Surgical complications
- Unhealthy cholesterol levels
- Urinary stress incontinence

The different types of cardiovascular disease are all interrelated and overlapping. **Arteriosclerosis** is a hardening of the arteries that can cut off bloodflow to the heart, causing a heart attack. When arteriosclerosis interrupts the flow of blood to the brain, it causes a **stroke**, also called a *brain attack*. Stroke affects about 4.5 million Americans each year.

Hardening of the arteries can also cause **high blood pressure**, or *hypertension*, a chronic elevation in the force your blood puts on artery walls. High blood pressure affects about 50 million Americans. Since it affects blood vessels throughout your entire body, it can lead to such varied problems as impaired vision and kidney damage. It's the most important risk factor for stroke, and it also can cause heart attack and congestive heart failure. Yet more terminology: **Congestive heart failure** means one side of your heart is so weak it can't pump out all the blood, so it tries to compensate by enlarging and pumping faster. If the failure occurs on the left side of the heart, fluid backs up into your lungs, causing shortness of breath, fatigue, and coughing—especially at night, and possibly expelling pink sputum. If it's on the right side, blood pools in your veins, and your feet, ankles, and legs begin to swell (a condition called *edema*). No matter which side of your heart is affected, the symptoms won't make you particularly popular on a Saturday night.

Since 1900, cardiovascular disease has been the number one killer of

Belly Busters

▶▶ "I grew up being known as The Fat Kid and had all the common nicknames, which ranged from Chunk to King Kong Bundy. Last September, [my doctor] informed me that my blood-sugar levels were high and that I had diabetes. . . . I thought to myself, 'There must be some mistake. I'm only 22. Older people get diabetes, not me!'

"After a restless night, I woke up determined to take control. I immediately cut off all sources of excess sugar and did 20 minutes of cardio every morning.

"After 7 months, I had gone from 206 pounds to 155. My blood sugar is down, and I have never felt this good and confident about myself. I don't ever have to worry about being called King Kong Bundy anymore." ◀◀

—MARK DOUANGCHANH
23, LOST 60 POUNDS

Americans. The only year it didn't top the list was 1918, when a flu epidemic killed 675,000 Americans and 20 million to 40 million people worldwide.

Lately, it's looked as if we're winning the war against heart disease. The death rate from heart attacks plunged from 400 per 100,000 people in 1970 to 170 per 100,000 in 1998. At the same time, the death rate from strokes decreased from 150 per 100,000 people to 60 per 100,000. The usual reasons cited are improved medical care, plus dietary changes that have reduced the amount of saturated fat in our diets from 16 to 12 percent. Today, we're more likely to consume poultry than red meat, low-fat milk than whole milk, margarine than butter, blah, blah, blah.

Behind these cheery statistics, however, is a grim reality: The rate at which Americans have heart attacks hasn't dropped as steeply—what we're really seeing is more people surviving

Belly Busters

▶▶▶ "In late December 2000, when my father was diagnosed with prostate cancer, I began to evaluate my own health and fitness. At the time, I was within weeks of my 37th birthday and weighed 241 pounds.

"When I went to my physician for a routine physical, my cholesterol count came in at 299. Both of my parents suffer from high cholesterol, and both have been on cholesterol medication for years. Because of the risk of heart disease associated with excess weight and high cholesterol, I decided to make some changes. I was determined to not only lose weight but also manage my cholesterol without the need for medication.

"At the beginning of the year, I was lucky to survive 15 minutes of cardio and a half-mile run. Now I'm down to 196 pounds, and I am at the point where I have recently registered to run in my first 10-K. When I had my cholesterol rechecked, it came in at 195.

"All told, I feel great and have made a commitment to maintain this healthy lifestyle. I cannot tell you how proud I feel when someone comments on my new look. That in itself is a tremendous motivation to continue." ◀◀

—JOE REPOSA
38, LOST 52 POUNDS

heart attacks, rather than substantially fewer people having them in the first place. And the decline in the death rates from heart attacks and strokes appears to be leveling off. So experts are increasingly worried that the obesity epidemic could reverse the gains we've seen in the fight against cardiovascular disease.

Few studies have examined the relationship between heart disease and waist circumference. It is known that a BMI over 25 gives you a one-in-four chance of having high blood pressure. (See the BMI chart on page 10 if you skipped past it the first time.) If you're an obese man—BMI over 30—the odds are greater than one in three that you have hypertension.

When researchers examined data from the Physicians' Health Study that has tracked 22,701 male physicians since 1982, they found that men whose waists measured more than 36.8 inches had a significantly elevated risk for two other types of heart disease: myocardial infarction and coronary revascularization. Men with the biggest bellies were at 60 percent higher risk.

IMPOTENCE

Yeah, we didn't want to talk about this one, either. But abdominal fat is as hard on your johnson as it is on your Jockeys. The stuff that gums up the blood vessels leading to your heart and brain also has a damming effect on your main vein. The result is softer erections or, in extreme cases, no erections.

CANCER

According to a Swedish study, the incidence of cancer among obese patients is 33 percent higher than among lean ones. And the World Health Organization estimates that up to one-third of cancers of the colon, kidney, and digestive tract are caused by being overweight and inactive. Overweight men also are at greater risk of developing cancers of the rectum and prostate.

Abdominal obesity is particularly dangerous since fat tissue spurs your body to produce hormones that prompt your cells to divide. Speeded-up cell division opens the window of opportunity for cancer-causing mutations to occur. Cancer cells that already exist get a greater chance to proliferate.

Several studies have linked abdominal obesity and colon cancer, and the association seems to be stronger in men than in women. When University of Pittsburgh researchers studied 5,849 people age 65 and older, they found that those with the highest waist circumferences had about twice the risk of developing colon cancer.

Obesity is also strongly associated with cancer of the esophagus. This is because overweight people are more likely to have gastroesophageal reflux disease, a condition in which stomach acid backs up into the esophagus and damages its lining. That damage causes speeded-up cell division, which then opens the door for cancer.

One study shows that excess weight accounts for 21 percent of kidney-cancer cases. Others show that heavier people are more prone to develop cancers of the gallbladder. Obesity also increases the risk of developing pancreatic cancer, the fifth-leading cause of cancer-related mortality in the United States.

Once cancer has developed, obesity makes it more difficult for doctors to calculate the most effective doses of radiation and chemotherapy. Studies also show that compared with thinner people, obese cancer patients tend to have worse outcomes and a harder time recovering.

SLEEP APNEA AND OTHER RESPIRATORY PROBLEMS

Apnea is a Greek word that means "without breath," making *obstructive sleep apnea* one of the most accurately descriptive terms we'll use in this chapter. (Okay, *high blood pressure* is pretty useful, too, since it describes a condition in which blood pressure is, uh, high.) The "obstructive" part comes in when soft tissue in the back of the throat collapses during sleep and blocks the airway.

When this happens, your brain signals you to wake up and start breathing again. Afterward, you probably won't fall back into a deep sleep right away. Even if you do, chances are you'll stop breathing again and start the whole process once more. When this occurs all night, every night, you're chronically groggy during your waking hours.

Sleep apnea becomes a social disease when your snorting and snoring and chronic waking make you impos-

Belly Busters

▶▶"I decided to diet last summer, after finally realizing that I was slowly killing myself. I could hear my heart beat when I lay down on the sofa."◀◀

—FRANK SERAFINI
30, LOST 80 POUNDS

sible to sleep with. And raising kids is tough enough when you're well-rested; imagine trying to do it when you're sleep deprived and short fused.

Another obvious side effect is that you perform poorly at work. Dozing off in meetings generally doesn't endear you to the boss and may prevent you from noticing when someone moves your cheese. Of course, that's assuming you even make it to work, since weight-related sleep apnea may make your commute more dangerous. When Stanford University researchers studied truck drivers, they found that overweight truckers had more than twice as many accidents per mile as thin ones. The researchers also noted that over half the accidents logged were caused by drivers who had sleep-disordered breathing.

Upper-body obesity is the most significant risk factor for obstructive sleep apnea. If you're extremely obese—BMI over 40—you're up to 30 times more likely than the general population to have sleep apnea. Obesity can impede the muscles that inflate and ventilate the lungs, forcing you to work harder to get enough air.

Belly fat also has a strong associa-tion with sleep apnea. When Australian researchers studied 313 patients with severe obesity, they found that 62 percent of those with a waist circumference of $49\frac{1}{2}$ inches or more had a serious sleep disturbance, compared to 28 percent of the obese men with smaller waists ($35\frac{1}{2}$ to 49 inches). In the general population, only 4 percent of men have sleep apnea.

The researchers noted that even the obese patients who were not diagnosed with sleep-disordered breathing reported increased sleep disturbances and daytime sleepiness. The most likely reason is that being overweight puts you at risk for a lot of conditions that rob you of a good night's rest, including asthma, gastroesophageal reflux (discussed above), and osteo-arthritis (discussed below).

When Dutch researchers studied 5,887 men, they found that even those whose waistlines measured a relatively modest 37 to 40 inches had a significantly increased risk of respiratory problems. Among them: wheezing without a cold, waking up with shortness of breath, coughing for more than 3 months, bringing up phlegm for more than 3 months, and shortness of breath when walking uphill or upstairs.

OSTEOARTHRITIS

Obese people are disproportionately prone to osteoarthritis, a degeneration of the cartilage that normally cushions joints and keeps bones from rubbing against each other. The heavier you are, the greater the chance that you'll rub your cartilage the wrong way. The knee is the most common problem area for heavyweights, but osteoarthritis also hits the hips and back. The result of damaged or worn-out cartilage is chronic pain and inflammation, leading to less activity.

As we've already seen, diminished activity means a greater chance you'll gain more weight and develop other conditions we describe in this chapter.

GALLBLADDER DISEASE

The gallbladder is a 4-inch-long sac of bile located between the liver and small intestine, and most of us go from cradle to grave without ever once thinking about it. Occasionally, too much cholesterol, one of the components of bile, builds up in the gallbladder and forms stones. Gallstones aren't a problem unless they block the ducts through which the bile flows. If that happens, jaundice, infection, and other nasty complications can ensue. Sometimes surgery is required.

As you've probably guessed by now, obesity triples your risk of developing gallstones. But here's something interesting and different: Rapid weight loss—due to stomach-stapling surgery or a super-low-calorie liquid diet, for example—also increases your chance of developing gallstones, as does yo-yo dieting, in which you lose and gain weight over and over.

CATARACTS AND
MACULAR DEGENERATION

All of us have our blind spots. No one likes to look in the mirror and honestly assess what's there. But when you're overweight or obese, your fat may prevent you from seeing yourself in the mirror at all.

New research from Harvard and Tufts Universities shows that belly fat increases your risk of developing two serious visual disorders: cataracts, a clouding of the lens that is the nation's leading cause of visual impairment; and macular degeneration, a progressive loss of central vision that's the leading cause of blindness.

When Harvard researchers examined data from over 17,000 of the male doctors in the Physicians' Health Study, they found that overweight men had a 20 percent higher risk of developing cataracts, while obese men had a 40 percent higher risk.

The eye's macula, at the center of the retina, contains the body's highest concentrations of lutein and zeaxanthin, two nutrients that protect the eyes by absorbing harmful blue light. (Bet you never knew shopping at Kmart posed such serious health risks.) When Tufts researchers analyzed belly fat, they found it soaks up at least

Belly Busters

▶▶"In 12 months, I lost 150 pounds. Things I don't miss are bleeding hemorrhoids, sleep apnea, always being tired, and, most of all, being large."◀◀

—MICHAEL GIBSON
34, LOST 143 POUNDS

twice as much lutein and zeaxanthin as fat in the hips and buttocks. Researchers suspect that belly fat may hog so much of these nutrients that not enough gets to the eyes.

GOUT

Back in the days when Henry VIII would down a couple of geese and maybe knock off a wife or two at a typical dinner, gout was a rich-man's disease. Only the powerful and affluent could eat enough fatty food to create the uric-acid crystals that settle in joints and create painful swelling and stiffness. (About half of gout cases affect the big toe.)

Today, given the proliferation of cheap fast food, gout has gone downmarket. Research has found that uric-acid levels are higher in overweight individuals. And abdominal obesity puts you at higher risk for a gouty toe than do other weight problems. When Japanese researchers studied 50 men ages 29 to 78, they found that those with the most visceral abdominal fat had the most uric acid in their bloodstreams. The bigger-bellied men also had the greatest difficulty eliminating uric acid from their bodies.

LIVER DISEASE

Being overweight is a risk factor for the development of alcohol-related liver diseases, including cirrhosis and acute hepatitis. And obesity is the most common cause of nonalcohol-related liver disease.

ACHES AND PAINS

When Dutch researchers studied 5,887 men ages 20 to 59, they found that those with waist circumferences above 40 inches were more than three times as likely to experience difficulty walking one block as men with waist circumferences smaller than 37 inches.

One possible reason: Big-bellied men are more likely to have chronic lower-back problems. They're also more likely to have Sever's disease, which causes excruciating heel pain.

Being obese also quadruples your risk of developing carpal tunnel syndrome, a painful hand-and-wrist condition that limits your ability to fill out the insurance forms to get treatment for your lower-back and heel pain. One study found that 70 percent of people with carpal tunnel syndrome were either overweight or obese.

Belly Busters

▶▶ "I maxed out at 291 pounds—even though I worked out routinely—and was just about the unhappiest man in the world due to my self-consciousness about my weight. My family doctor suggested that if I didn't lose a large amount of weight soon, I wouldn't live to see my grandchildren.

"I went on a diet-and-exercise program with the guidance of a dietitian, a gastroenterologist, and my family doctor. Now, 15 years later, I weigh 186 pounds." ◀◀

—KEN ARMSTRONG
51, LOST 107 POUNDS

Belly Off SUCCESS STORY

Life of a Salesman

LIFE IN THE FAT LANE

As a teenager, Gil Craig ran a 4:38 mile, weighed 115 pounds, and was turned down for a factory job because he was too skinny.

Then he grew up—and out. Marriage, fatherhood, and a demanding sales job consumed his life. "I stopped exercising and ate the wrong kinds of foods," he says.

By age 54, Craig weighed 230 pounds and wore size-44 pants. His once well-defined chin and jaw had merged into a turkey neck that sank straight into his shoulders. "I was a fat alcoholic," he says.

Portents of disaster surrounded him. His mother had developed diabetes in middle age and lived a miserable life until she died of cancer at 80. His brother had been a heavy drinker who died of liver failure at 50.

Craig made several halfhearted attempts to get in shape. "Once I even joined a gym. But I didn't like it, so I dropped out and never went back."

His belly, swollen by burgers and booze, made him feel ashamed, inferior, and invisible.

In late 1999, Craig applied for life insurance and flunked the physical. "I brushed it off and went on with my life as usual," he says.

Which is to say, he remained a mess. When he looked down, he couldn't see his feet . . . or his penis, which he nicknamed Willie. Willie increasingly became a stranger to Craig, who had no desire for sex. It got to the point that Willie was summoned for duty just once a month—the erectile equivalent of an army reservist.

Craig also had problems with frequent urination, excessive thirst, shortness of breath, and insomnia. His wife, Lynn, a registered nurse, talked him into seeing a doctor, who found that he had high blood pressure, high cholesterol, high blood sugar, and a liver-enzyme abnormality. He

was also diagnosed with type-2, or adult-onset, diabetes.

After a lifetime of avoiding medications, Craig was suddenly on three prescription drugs.

THE TURNING POINT

One evening that winter, Craig checked into a hotel room after another long day on the road. "As I stood buck-naked in front of a full-length mirror, I stopped to stare at the monument I had built," he says.

Then he looked at his row of medications and vowed that he would not go down the same road that his mother and brother had.

(continued)

Name: GIL CRAIG
Date of Birth: October 1945
Residence: Glassboro, New Jersey
Occupation: Salesman
Height: 5 foot 8

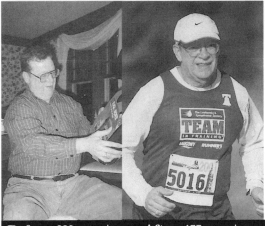

Before: 230 pounds   **After:** 177 pounds

THE PLAN OF ATTACK

When Craig got home, he dusted off an unused treadmill and climbed aboard. During his first session, he could barely last 20 minutes. "But I stuck with it and gradually increased my speed and distance," he says.

He began eating better, and the weight started to drop off. "I noticed a 5-pound drop here, a 5-pound drop there," he says. "When I broke the 200 barrier, it was like, 'Wow, this is something!'"

In the spring of 2000, Craig began walking every morning on a half-mile track. When he underwent his first physical since getting in shape, he weighed 185 pounds and had normal blood pressure, blood sugar, and blood cholesterol. His doctor told him to stop taking his medications.

With a renewed spirit, Craig began training for a 1-mile run. "I completed it in 7 minutes, 24 seconds," he says. "It was a far cry from my high school time, but I figured, 'I'll take it.'"

By the time he was able to run a 5-K, he was a changed man. "My beer belly and turkey neck had disappeared," he says. Six months into his program, he weighed 165 pounds and wore size-34 pants.

He kept running outdoors even after winter arrived. He also began using a weight set that his son-in-law, a body-builder, had given him. "I started with the basic press, curl, bench press, and reverse curl," he says. "I combined my front leg lifts with situps. After several weeks, I started to see fat change to muscle."

LIFE IN THE FIT LANE

As Craig's body changed, so did his attitude. He and his wife joined a choir. He became a youth basketball coach. Even his productivity picked up. "I took a poor-performing territory and increased sales so it's now one of the best territories," he says.

Although Craig has incorporated more strength training into his routine—adding 10 to 15 pounds of muscle while maintaining his 34-inch waist—he figures he spends 60 percent of his exercise time on cardiovascular exercise and just 40 percent with the weights. "I run almost every day," he says.

He doesn't consider himself a dieter—just a smarter eater. He eliminated fast foods, snack foods, and fatty foods such as eggs, bacon, and sausage. He ate oatmeal and a banana for breakfast; a piece of fruit, yogurt, or a can of tuna for lunch; and whatever he wanted for dinner.

"If it's red meat, I don't care," he says. "That's my reward."

He also cut back on his drinking. "Now I try to limit myself to three beers," he says.

Craig worked up to a half-marathon, then a full marathon. Before running in the Philadelphia Marathon in 2001, he saw the same doctor who had diagnosed him with diabetes. "He was totally amazed," says Craig. "He just looked at my chart, shook his head, and called me his healthiest patient."

HIS TIPS

REORDER YOUR PRIORITIES. "It used to be that my whole life revolved around work and making money. My job controlled my life. I needed to break out of a life that was killing me."

LIVE FOR TODAY. "I could be doing all this and be dead tomorrow from an aneurysm. But today I'm going to enjoy my body. The years I have left are going to be mine. All mine."

Belly
Sabotage

THE FIRST DISAPPOINTMENT A GIRL EXPERIENCES IN LIFE, SOMEONE once wrote, is realizing she'll never be a princess. In theory, she gets over this sometime in junior high. The first disappointment a guy experiences is realizing he'll never quarterback the Packers. He gets over this shortly after his stock options vest.

For a guy trying to lose excess weight, an even more enduring disappointment is the idea that his genes prevent him from ever being lean. And we aren't going to yank you on this one: Research does show a genetic component to the way your body packs on the pounds.

Here are some conclusions researchers have drawn.

▶ Twenty-five to 40 percent of obesity is determined by genetics, according to a 1996 review by Claude Bouchard, Ph.D., one of the world's most respected obesity researchers.

▶ Studies of identical twins who were systematically overfed showed that heredity does influence how much weight is gained from overeating, how much of that weight is fat, and what percentage of fat versus carbohydrates is metabolized for energy over the course of a day. The pairs of twins who gained the most

Belly Busters

▶▶"Easter of 2000, when I went home to Mom's for the annual feast of ham and deviled eggs, the realization that I was part of a fat family hit home. My mother, God bless her, is 5 foot 8 and weighs over 200 pounds; and my brother, 5 years my senior, is in excess of 300. Both have serious health problems. That afternoon, as I looked in the mirror, reality kicked in: I looked like a blimp.

"On the way home, I told my wife that enough was enough, and this excess baggage had to go. Interestingly enough, she was having the same thoughts about my situation. She said she loved me very much, but she didn't want me to turn out like the rest of my family: obese and plagued with medical problems."◀◀

—JAMES GORDON
44, LOST 60 POUNDS

weight also gained the highest percentage of fat—up to 80 percent. And those who gained the least weight gained the lowest percentage of fat—about one-third.

▶ When identical twins were given exercise programs that burned 58,000 calories, similar patterns emerged. Since a pound of fat contains 3,500 calories, that much exercise should produce weight loss of 16½ pounds. But the amount of weight lost by the study subjects varied from as little as 2.2 pounds to as much as 17.6 pounds, with each twin losing about the same amount as his sibling. (Wouldn't you love to be a twin who lost *more* weight than you and your brother should have? And how much would it suck to be the one of the poor guys who did enough work to lose 16½ pounds but lost only the equivalent of a really good steak dinner?)

▶ A 1999 study in the *American Journal of Human Biology* found that 50 to 55 percent of your abdominal fat can be attributed to a genetic link.

So let's not sugarcoat it: Your genes do influence how much weight you gain from overeating, how much weight you lose from exercise, and how much of that weight is concentrated in your belly. In fact, Bouchard found that genetics influences even your choices of fat versus carbohydrate foods, as well as the amount of alcohol you consume.

Knowing this doesn't really help you much, however. You could hope that someday scientists will find a way to manipulate your troublemaking genes and change your pot luck. But even if they do, you'll still have to deal with the other 50 percent of the reasons why you store fat preferentially in your midsection.

Fittingly, those other sources of your android fat begin with the letter A: anger, anxiety, and alcohol.

THE GROWLING BELLY

In a Penn State study of middle-age and older men, printed in 1999 in *Obesity Research*, the angriest, most anxious, and most cynical ones also turned out to have the most belly fat, as determined by waist-hip ratio. Anger was a gut expander in both middle-age and older men, while anxiety and cynicism were associated with abdominal fat only in middle age men.

The culprit in all three cases seems to be cortisol, a hormone produced by your tiny adrenal glands, which sit atop your kidneys. In this case, bad things come from small packages.

THE ANTI-TESTOSTERONE

Like testosterone, cortisol is a steroid hormone. Its similarity to the muscle-building T-dog pretty much ends there. While testosterone is your belly-off ally, cortisol may have contributed to your gut getting there in the first place. Here's how: When you're under high levels of physical or psychological stress—when you're overtraining, starving yourself, or simply stressed out—your adrenal glands release an overabundance of cortisol, setting off a cascade of gut-growing effects. First, cortisol stimulates your appetite: Suddenly, you can't drive by a Dunkin' Donuts without devouring a half-dozen Boston creams. Cortisol triggers your hunger by turning off your body's built-in satiety switch. Your brain never gets the signal that you're full, so you keep eating.

Cortisol also activates the fat-gathering enzyme lipoprotein lipase, which in turn rounds up the excess calories from all those doughnuts and shuttles them directly to your belly-fat stores. Your gut's visceral fat has a greater abundance of cortisol receptors than any other part of your body, and these receptors act like magnets, attracting the cortisol and the fat that its enzyme pal rounds up.

To make matters worse, stress also raises your blood-glucose level. Several processes lead to this blood-sugar spike, including cortisol's mobilization of glucose from the liver. What's more, if you're under extreme stress for a long duration, the constant high levels of cortisol can lead to insulin resistance, elevated blood pressure, and high cholesterol.

Cortisol's negative effects don't end there. It actually suppresses your testosterone levels, which spells disaster for the guy trying to put on muscle. As your cortisol levels rise, your T levels plummet—and so does your ability to build new muscle. Instead of going to the gym, you might as well head home and catch *Three Stooges* reruns. At least

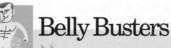

Belly Busters

▶▶ "I can now look in the mirror with more self-respect and pride in myself. I went from 240 pounds and a 38-inch waist to 190-to-195 pounds and a 32-to-33-inch waist. I can see abs I never dreamed I would see, and my confidence has increased considerably.

"I now get compliments from family and friends. But the best payoff is knowing I did it and now I can stick to it." ◀◀

—STERLING RASKIE
25, LOST 55 POUNDS

you could start to lower your stress level by getting a few laughs.

In times of severe, prolonged stress (such as if your plane crashed in the Andes and you were close to starvation), cortisol actually signals your body to break down its own muscle tissue. (Now *that's* the kind of cannibalism they should have shown in the movie *Alive*. Truly scary stuff.)

To determine whether stress-trig-gered cortisol could be taking a toll on *your* body, look for these signs: irritability, sleeping or memory problems, or a feeling of constant tiredness and near-exhaustion.

ONE IS THE DEADLIEST NUMBER

Although the amount of cortisol released matters, the biggest problem associated with abdominal obesity is an erratic and upredictable cortisol

---

Exercise: The Ultimate Happy Pill

You've probably heard that regular exercise relieves anxiety and depression. But until recently, researchers weren't exactly sure why.

In 2001, British researchers presented a study showing that exercise elevates your body's levels of phenylethylamine, a brain chemical linked to energy, mood, and attention. During the study, 20 healthy young men ran on a treadmill for 30 minutes. Afterward, researchers took urine samples and found that the average concentration of phenylacetic acid, a metabolized derivative of phenylethylamine, increased by 77 percent.

Since the chemical is similar to amphetamines, the researchers speculated it could be responsible for the so-called runner's high.

Other research shows that people with depression or bipolar disorder (manic depression) have lower-than-normal levels of phenylacetic acid in their urine.

Moderate exercise can slow production of the stress hormone cortisol. Many studies have shown that moderate exercise also reduces stress, improves mood, builds self-esteem, and reprograms your brain for optimism instead of pessimism.

As your fitness level in-creases, so do the psychological benefits. Texas A&M researchers tested 15 volunteers in a 9-day adventure program that included such activities as whitewater canoeing, rock climbing, and hiking while carrying heavy backpacks (35 to 45 percent of each subject's body weight). The fittest participants were not only better equipped for the physical challenges but also were better prepared for the mental and emotional stress. Urine tests confirmed that they had lower levels of cortisol and two other stress hormones—epinephrine and norepinephrine—than less-fit participants.

release that occurs when least expected.

One of the best predictors of abnormal cortisol release is isolation. For example, baby laboratory rats that aren't nurtured by Ma Rat end up with more of the hormones that trigger cortisol and fewer of the brain receptors that would blunt its effects. At least one study has shown that humans raised in isolation—in this case, Romanian orphans—have abnormal cortisol function.

It's too soon to know whether these children will grow up to have high levels of abdominal obesity. But it seems possible, given the findings of a Swedish study published in 1996 in the *International Journal of Obesity*. In that study of 1,040 middle-age men, the ones with high waist-hip ratios were more likely to be divorced, have an unsatisfying social life, live alone in poor housing conditions, earn a lower income, and have more problems at work. (Middle-age men who were overweight without pronounced abdominal fat tended to be married or cohabiting, and had relatively few problems at work.) The big-bellied, isolated guys also showed more symptoms of depression and anxiety than other middle-age men.

Of course, you have to wonder: Does depression cause a big gut, or does a big gut cause depression? Researchers are split on this one.

One theory suggests that an impaired quality of life might cause abdominal obesity because of increased

Belly Busters

▶▶"At one point in time, mirrors and scales were two things that haunted me. I never wanted to face the mirror to see my image or step on the scale to see the numbers.

"Now, I'm in the best shape I've ever been in, and I can say that the fat kid I once was is no longer. This summer when I'm at the pool, I will do the one thing I have always wanted to do: take my shirt off and feel good about it."◀◀

—JONATHAN HEATON
23, LOST 95 POUNDS

cortisol secretion. In a 1999 study published in *Obesity Research*, however, Penn State University researchers surveyed 1,392 men and women and found that depression was a predictor of abdominal obesity only in middle-age women.

Another chicken-and-egg question arises when looking at the connection between depression and diabetes type 2. We know for certain that overeating and avoiding exercise can be symptoms of depression. They also can set you up for diabetes type 2. Furthermore, depression can cause insulin resistance. And insulin resistance, as you know, is a precursor of diabetes.

When Washington University School of Medicine researchers reviewed 42 studies exploring the link between depression and diabetes, they found that people with diabetes are *twice* as likely as nondiabetics to be depressed. In most cases, depression predated diabetes.

Another Washington University School of Medicine study concluded that depressed diabetics don't control their blood sugar as effectively as nondepressed diabetics. Consequently, they suffer higher rates of heart, kidney, and eye complications.

No matter which comes first—the belly or the beast of depression—it's crucial to treat depression if you have it. Unfortunately, some of the most popular antianxiety and antidepressant drugs have brutal complications. Many guys on paroxetine (Paxil) and fluoxetine (Prozac) gain weight and, even more humiliating, experience erectile dysfunction. Nothing punctuates a problem like finding that your exclamation point has turned into a comma.

Though the impotence caused by these drugs is the most frightening side effect, it tends to be temporary. It's also the type of problem a shrink takes seriously. No doctor wants to alleviate a guy's depression at the expense of his manhood.

Antidepressants' relationship to weight gain is more puzzling. Some people lose weight when taking antidepressants; others gain. Doctor and patient will have to find one that will relieve depression without causing intolerable weight gain.

BELLYING UP TO THE BAR

Our final belly bomber is the least surprising. Whatever you call it—beer gut, Bud tumor, Guinness goiter—you associate a bigger waistline with excess alcohol consumption.

It seems that alcohol actually encourages your body to burn less fat. That's what Swiss researchers discovered when they gave eight healthy men enough alcohol to exceed their daily calorie requirements by 25 percent. (If you normally eat 3,000 calories a day, it would take just over five 150-calorie beers to exceed your intake by 25 percent.) Turns out, the booze impaired the men's ability to burn fat by as much as 36 percent.

The only surprising fact is that chronic heavy-duty drinkers are usually leaner than moderate drinkers.

When researchers compared 34 alcoholics with 43 control subjects, they found that the two groups weighed the same. The alcoholics actually had a slightly lower amount of overall body fat.

They did, however, have more visceral abdominal fat the fat close to their livers, which were already compromised by chronic, heavy alcohol consumption. The researchers

Belly Busters

▶▶"Ever since I lost the weight, I've noticed that my body fits into more designer clothing and I'm more confident at my workplace."◀◀

—ARMANDO SPATARO
23, LOST 55 POUNDS

concluded that heavy drinkers with potbellies have an even greater likelihood of developing alcoholic liver disease.

To us, the weirdest thing about liquor is that in small amounts it's clearly associated with positive health outcomes, while in larger quantities it's devastating. For example, the Honolulu Heart Study of 8,006 men showed that one or two drinks a day was associated with a 54 percent decrease in heart-attack deaths. An Australian review of more than 2,700 studies on alcohol and health showed that men who average one drink a day have a 16 percent lower death rate than abstainers.

Statistics like those probably make you want to grab a beer. Don't pop that top just yet—the cheery news about moderate alcohol consumption has to be put into context.

First off, alcohol's heart-protective benefits might not kick in until you're way past legal drinking age. When researchers calculated the years of life lost and gained in England and Wales as a result of drinking alcohol, they found that the most gains were seen among men over age 55. For maximum benefits, they concluded that men should not even begin drinking moderate amounts of alcohol until after age 34.

On an even more depressing note, the researchers found that in one year alone, alcohol robbed English- and Welshmen under age 44 of a combined total of 75,000 years of life. The

Belly Busters

▶▶ "Sorry, guys, you gotta cut down on the booze. For real. That stuff just makes you fat. You can enjoy a beer with the boys, but you can't drink a six pack on a regular basis and expect to be thin." ◀◀

—MARK OHLINGER
31, LOST 60 POUNDS

damage resulted mostly from alcohol-related traffic accidents, suicides, and liver disease.

Regardless of your age, alcohol's health benefits vanish once you put away more than 3 drinks a day. When researchers tracked 12,261 middle-age participants for 3 to 6 years in the Atherosclerosis Risk in Communities Study, they found that men who consumed more than 21 drinks a week (more than 3 per day) were 50 percent more likely to develop diabetes type 2 than men who consumed fewer than 1 drink a week. The diabetes risk was even higher among men who drank hard liquor. Men who consumed more than 14 drinks of spirits a week were 80 percent more likely to develop diabetes than men who drank only beer or wine.

Alcohol in any form can turn your $33\frac{1}{3}$-inch waistline into an extended dance remix. When French researchers studied the drinking habits of 1,778 men ages 35 to 64, they found that wine and spirits were just as likely as beer to cause a beer belly. The more the men drank of *any* kind

Sweet Spirits

A craving for alcohol might actually be a craving for sugar. When you consume alcohol or sugar, your body deals with those calories first. Just as alcohol could immediately take the edge off a stressful situation, a sugary snack might give you an instant lift.

One Duke University study found that people who quit drinking craved sweets and fats.

Another study showed that laboratory rats drank less alcohol when they were fed chocolate.

So there's just one more reason why you'll drink less when the happy-hour special is a chocolate martini.

of alcohol, the fatter they got around their middles. Your beer gut could just as easily be a Burgundy belly or tequila tumor.

While alcohol expands your waist, it also shrinks your thigh and gluteal muscles. Those are the biggest muscles on your body, so a heavy drinker can lose as much as 20 percent of his entire muscle mass. Some experts believe the culprit behind this carnage is, once again, the stress hormone cortisol.

In fact, the effects of alcohol and cortisol are nearly identical: Both decrease protein synthesis (the process that causes your muscles to grow bigger and stronger) and reduce levels of testosterone and insulin-like growth factor (another muscle-building hormone).

Exercise doesn't seem to offer protection from these ravages. A small study showed that cortisol levels rose 61 percent when participants drank alcohol after a strength-training session.

He Let Out His Inner Self

LIFE IN THE FAT LANE

While growing up in Montreal, Geoffrey White fought a seesaw battle against his belly. Soon after he started college (or "entered university," as they say in Canada), it appeared that his belly had won.

His social life was a disappointment, and he sought solace in suds and fast food. "Big Macs at 2:00 in the morning aren't especially good for you," he says.

By the time White graduated in 1998, he weighed more than 350 pounds and wore size-48 pants. The excess weight strained his back, knees, and feet, and he had shockingly little endurance. "Walking upstairs, I felt really out of breath," he says.

He also perspired a lot, which made him feel even more self-conscious—especially around women.

During summer breaks, White served in the army reserves, an experience that taught him to hate exercise. "I didn't like the discipline. I didn't like being forced to exercise," he says. "I

shouldn't have been there in the first place because I was so out of shape."

He resumed his sedentary ways as soon as he returned to school each fall. And he dealt with his frustrating social life as he always had: by stuffing his face. "It became a vicious cycle."

THE TURNING POINT

In some respects, White was lucky. He didn't develop diabetes, heart disease, high blood pressure, or any of the other ailments that often strike young, overweight guys.

But White's emotional pain was intense. "I was so unhappy with my looks and my body," he says. "I just felt unhealthy."

Fresh out of college and ready to start work in the corporate-communications field, White moved in with a buddy in Toronto. The date was January 1, 1999.

White knew there was a small

gym in the basement of his apartment building. So, like countless other guys before him, he made a resolution to get fit.

The difference is, he kept it.

THE PLAN OF ATTACK

White immediately placed himself on a strict, low-fat diet. "I cut out the fat, the grease, the potatoes, and the volume," he says. "I also cut out the night eating, which I'm convinced was a major problem for me."

During the first year, he subsisted largely on a diet of chicken,

(continued)

Name: GEOFFREY WHITE
Date of Birth: September 1975
Residence: Toronto
Occupation: Corporate communications
Height: 6 foot 4

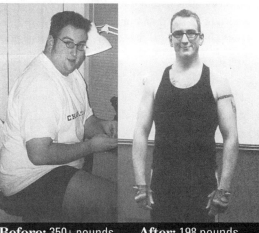

Before: 350+ pounds   **After:** 198 pounds

turkey sandwiches, rice, and vegetables. From the beginning, however, he refused to eliminate two of his favorite indulgences: beer and soda. "I'm living my bachelor years now," he reasoned.

In the basement gymnasium, he worked out on a stairclimber 6 days a week. "Then I became smarter about what I was doing and began wearing a heart-rate monitor and running on a treadmill," he says.

He also embraced other lifestyle changes such as walking to work and taking stairs instead of escalators.

The fat melted away. Within a year, White had lost nearly 100 pounds, going from more than 350 pounds to 276 pounds.

Along the way, he met a girlfriend. She was a good cheerleader—and more important, she recognized that there was more to White than the way he looked. "She saw me for my inner self," he says.

The relationship didn't last, but it was exactly the kind of boost White needed. More than ever, he was determined to get in shape.

During the second year, White added strength training to his exercise routine. Soon, it ac-counted for 50 percent of the time he spent in the gym.

The results surprised him.

"I swear by the weight training," he says. "In terms of weight loss and toning, that's where I noticed the biggest difference. Now it makes up almost 90 percent of my gym time."

Two years into his program, he was down to 195 pounds and size-34 pants—a stunning, 155-pound drop. "I lost a whole Backstreet Boy," he says.

LIFE IN THE FIT LANE

While White enjoyed increased attention from women, he found that the greatest rewards came from within.

"The greatest thing ever was doing a chinup for the first time in my life," he says. After accomplishing this feat of strength in 2000, White's self-confidence soared. Then came more achievements that he had never thought possible: dips, climbing the stairs of the 1,800-foot CN Tower, pushups and situps by the dozen.

"Although I'm not a very athletic or team-sport-oriented guy, I know there's not a single sport I would shy away from because I'm not fit enough," he says.

Take indoor rock climbing, for example—an activity that White took up during the summer of 2001. "That's something a 350-pound guy never does," he says.

Scaling walls not only presented a physical challenge but also helped him conquer a lifelong fear of heights. Soon, he plans to start scaling rocks in the great outdoors.

There have been some bumps along the way, including two hernias—one of which required surgery. Still, White would rather be a thin guy with reparable problems than a fat guy with irreparable ones.

"I'm in control of how long I will live now," he says. "Even though a bus may hit me tomorrow, at least I'm not going to die because I smoked or drank too much or ate too much fat."

HIS TIPS

SNACK SMART. "If the need for junk food arises, make smart choices like eating licorice."

INDULGE SENSIBLY. "Although I still eat a lot of chicken, rice, and vegetables, I'm not against red meat or bacon and eggs on the weekend, or beer or anything like that. I need those sorts of indulgences to keep me sane."

CHAPTER

5

Defusing
the Danger

NUTRITIONIST NANCY CLARK, R.D., OF BROOKLINE, MASSACHUSETTS, once said something that may resonate with you if you've ever fallen off the diet-and-exercise wagon: "If you rely on willpower to lose weight, you're defeated before you've begun."

Sure, some people can stick with extremely restrictive diets or brutal exercise programs for a week or two. Maybe some can do it even longer. But in the long run, your plan won't work if it depends on making you miserable. If you starve yourself, your body's needs will eventually overpower your will to deny them. If you exercise to excess, your body will eventually break down, preventing you from exercising at all. And if you try to do both, your body will break down even faster.

Weight loss works best if you have two elements: a diet you can live with and an exercise program that allows you to work out consistently.

EATING LESS
VERSUS MOVING MORE

An intriguing Dutch study published in 2001 in the *American Journal of Clinical Nutrition* found that when obese men were

43

put on a diet without exercise, they burned a lower percentage of fat for energy. The researchers put 40 obese men (average age 39) on a low-calorie diet. Half of the subjects also did low-intensity exercise, while the other half remained sedentary. Both groups lost the same amount of fat—about 30 pounds—in 10 weeks. Two weeks after the diet ended, the non-exercising group was burning less fat for energy than they had before the study.

The implication of this is huge: Weight loss achieved by diet alone could signal your body to burn less fat for energy. Even light regular exercise counteracts this decline in fat metabolism.

A 2000 study in *Annals of Internal Medicine* looked at the diet-and-exercise question a different way: The researchers wanted to know what effect different strategies had on visceral abdominal fat and some of the associated health problems. They divided 52 obese men into four groups: diet-induced weight loss, exercise-induced weight loss, exercise without weight

loss, and none of the above (the control group). (Actually, the study started with 101 participants, but only 52 finished, showing that even in a clinical setting, the weight-loss-program dropout rate is around 50 percent.) After 3 months, the guys in the two weight-loss groups had each dropped about 16½ total pounds, with the exercisers each losing almost ½ pound more, on average. Both groups lost similar amounts of visceral abdominal fat: about 2 pounds per guy, which was about one-quarter of the visceral fat each began with.

But the exercise-induced weight-loss guys each lost about 5 pounds more fat and 1 pound less muscle. And while both weight-loss groups saw their metabolisms slow down as a result of the lost muscle, the dieters got the worse end of the deal: Each dieter's metabolism slowed by about 212 calories a day, while each exerciser's metabolism ended up only 126 calories a day slower.

(Important point: The exercise was aerobic—walking or running on a treadmill—and the diet was low-fat and carbohydrate-heavy. Change the exercise to weight training and the diet to one with more fat and protein and fewer carbohydrates, and you'd probably see increased muscle mass and metabolisms in the exercise group. But we'll talk more about that in later chapters.)

Right here, you have a pretty good argument for diet-plus-exercise over diet alone. But this study also had a

Belly Busters

▶▶"I didn't weigh myself very much at first. I didn't have a scale at home, and still don't. I kept track of my weight loss by how my pants fit."◀◀

—MARK OHLINGER
31, LOST 60 POUNDS

group that exercised while increasing their daily calories by about 700. Interestingly, these guys each lost, on average, about a pound of visceral abdominal fat, which was about 15 percent of the amount each started with. They each gained about a pound of muscle. Each guy's metabolism increased by an average of 371 calories burned a day.

Another interesting finding was that insulin sensitivity improved in both weight-loss groups as well as in the exercise-without-weight-loss group.

We can extrapolate three solid conclusions from these two studies.

1. Diet alone will help you lose visceral fat and improve your health, but will also slow your metabolism and signal your body to burn more carbohydrates for energy—a prescription for weight regain. Another, very scary study in *Obesity Research* looked at people who had each lost 14 pounds on a 28-day crash diet. Five years later, they had regained all the weight, with a twist: All the new weight was fat, whereas they'd originally lost a combination of fat and muscle. And their health had deteriorated in multiple ways, including increased insulin resistance and higher LDL cholesterol.

Another drawback of diet alone is that in order to lose weight, you have to restrict calories more severely than you would if you were also exercising.

2. Exercise alone will also help you lose your gut and improve insulin sensitivity while increasing your metabo-

Belly Busters

▶▶"I recently lost 40 pounds by following what I call the Fitness Magazine Diet. The diet was created by reading every magazine regarding health, exercise, and fitness I could get my hands on, for several months on end. I would cut out any article related to eating, working out, running, tips, food suggestions, supplementation, motivation, etcetera. If I read similar tips in different magazines, I would make that tip part of my lifestyle."◀◀

—RAFFAEL BORELLI
34

lism. As long as you keep exercising, this should maintain past weight loss and prevent future weight gain. However, you have to spend more time exercising than you would if you also had a controlled diet.

3. Exercise plus diet appears to be the ticket: You reap all the benefits of each without resorting to extremes in either.

THE VIRTUOUS SPIRAL
The key to making diet and exercise work over the long term? Finding a way to enjoy it.

To see how this plays out, let's look at a study published in *Obesity Research* in 2000 that surveyed a group of 931 people, including 173 men, who had lost and kept off at least 30 pounds. The researchers divided the subjects into three groups: those who had maintained their weight loss for 2 to 3 years, those who had maintained

Belly Busters

▶▶"I plan what I eat (six meals per day), and I know what I am going to accomplish in the gym before I walk through the doors."◀◀

—HOBIE JONES
44, LOST 28 POUNDS

for 3 to 6 years, and those who had kept it off for 6 or more years.

They found that the groups were similar in many respects: They all derived about the same amount of pleasure from exercise, diet, and weight maintenance. More than 70 percent in each group weighed themselves regularly and bought books or magazines related to diet and exercise (thanks, guys).

But here's the cool finding in this study: "Subjects with longer durations reported that significantly less effort was required to diet and to maintain weight and that less attention was required to maintain weight."

The people who maintained weight loss the longest also lost the most weight and weighed less, on average, than the others.

When you add it up, you see that the greatest weight loss—and the greatest success in maintaining it—is associated with the least effort. That doesn't mean *no* effort, of course. It just means that the longer you keep weight off, the easier it gets.

It's what we call a *virtuous spiral.* Here's how it works.

You find a diet that works for you, based on foods you enjoy.

You develop an exercise program that works for you, including hard, endorphin-stimulating workouts two or three times a week. (Although you could find the right workout before the right diet, or get lucky enough to hit both at the same time.)

You turn your effort into a hobby, weighing yourself regularly and reading books and magazines that show you newer, better, or just more interesting ways to eat good food and get in productive workouts.

You realize that, in order to eat better and exercise consistently, you need to clean up other areas of your life. You avoid situations that you know will set back your progress.

Your exercise may help you sleep better, so you develop a more regular sleep schedule: in bed at the same time each night, up at the same time each morning.

You start feeling better about yourself and your life, since exercise has a well-known mood-improving effect.

When all parts of the spiral are working for you, you aren't depriving yourself. You aren't relying on willpower to get through the day without a run to Krispy Kreme. You're enjoying yourself. You look good, you feel good, and you can't imagine going back to the life in which you didn't look and feel this way.

That's what the Belly-Off Program is all about.

He Defanged His Sweet Tooth

LIFE IN THE FAT LANE

Johnny L. Scott never thought of himself as a fat man. He lifted weights, after all, and figured his workouts gave him the freedom to eat whatever he wanted. "I love sweets," he says. "And I used to drink an enormous amount of soda—at least four or five cans a day."

Scott's cravings for Coca-Cola, Krispy Kreme doughnuts, chocolate, and fried foods inevitably took their toll. Between the ages of 24 and 34, his once rail-thin frame increased from 139 pounds to 208 pounds.

Although he felt like a stuffed sausage in his business suits, it wasn't enough to scare him away from comfort foods. "I didn't worry about how much I ate," he says.

Nor was he especially concerned about his high cholesterol. He figured he was still young enough to get it under control before it did too much damage.

What did bother him was his increasing fatigue. At 34, he felt as wiped out as an old man.

"I was always tired," he says. "I'd get up in the morning and feel tired. All day long, I'd feel tired. I knew something was wrong."

THE TURNING POINT

In December 1999, Scott learned that something was *seriously* wrong. A routine physical showed that he had a fasting blood-sugar level of 265. That's three times higher than normal—a sure sign he had diabetes.

"No one in my family had diabetes, so I was really shocked," he says. "I was in denial, wondering 'How could this happen to me?' Because I always exercised, I didn't think it *would* happen to me."

A month later, he had fewer doubts about his diagnosis. Plagued by constant thirst and emergency trips to the restroom, he also found that his beloved sweets were bringing on killer headaches.

"It was like, 'Oh yeah, I guess it really is a lot more serious than I thought,'" he says.

After a blood test confirmed he had type-2, or adult-onset, diabetes, he learned everything he could about the disease and its complications, including heart disease, vision loss, nerve damage, limb amputations, and premature death. "That's enough to scare you," he says.

He realized he had a choice: either take control of diabetes or let it take control of him.

THE PLAN OF ATTACK

Since Scott loathes needles, he hated the idea that he might eventually have to take insulin shots. So he resolved to control

(continued)

Name: JOHNNY L. SCOTT
Date of Birth: July 1965
Residence: Rancho Cucamonga, California
Occupation: Finance manager, United Parcel Service
Height: 5 foot 10

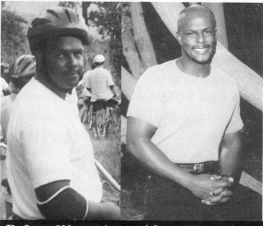

Before: 208 pounds   **After:** 175 pounds

his blood sugar naturally with diet and exercise.

His first step was ditching sweets, sodas, and fried foods, and switching to a diet rich in fresh fruits, vegetables, and grilled chicken and fish.

"You can adjust to it," he says of his healthier eating habits. "If you make it a part of your life and stick with it, you don't have the same types of cravings that you had before."

He found his weight-lifting routine wasn't enough to control his weight and blood sugar, so he began running every weekday.

In 6 months, he lost 33 pounds.

Intent on pummeling his pot-belly into submission, he performed 100 situps in the morning and another 100 at bedtime.

His blood-sugar and cholesterol levels plummeted to normal levels. He takes no medications and envisions a future free of needles.

Since diabetes is a relentless foe, however, Scott realizes that he can't ever drop his guard. He knows it would be suicidal to go back to his old ways. "That's why I take care of myself," he says. "I watch what I eat, exercise, and stay in very good shape."

LIFE IN THE FIT LANE

Scott now recognizes that his weight had endangered his health, ruined his physique, and made him old before his time.

With his diabetes under control, he has energy to burn. "It makes a huge difference not to be tired all day," he says. In the mornings, Scott gets up with enough vigor to do 200 situps before breakfast, followed by another 200 situps before he goes to work. This has helped him to maintain and sculpt his 29-inch waist.

Scott is especially happy with the more youthful, energetic image he presents at work. "When you're looking better in your suits, you're feeling better about yourself," he says. "You get more favorable responses from people, including, I should say, females."

Though diabetes prevents him from taking cheat days with his diet, he does drink a can or two of diet soda a day to satisfy his sweet tooth. On very rare occasions, he treats himself to a piece of chocolate. "If I eat something sweet, then I can't eat something else," he says. "That's what I have to do so that my blood sugar doesn't fluctuate."

Scott doesn't take all the credit for his transformation. As a devout Christian, he believes he received a crucial assist from the Big Guy.

"My belief in Jesus Christ definitely helped me," he says. "Without it, it would have been extremely difficult for me, especially in the beginning. There were times when I thought, 'I don't even know if I can do this. . . . Do I really want to change my lifestyle? Is it going to be too difficult for me to change?'"

In the end, it doesn't matter who gets the credit: Scott has proved that it is possible to change.

HIS TIPS

PUSH AND PULL. "When I lift weights, I'll do pushing exercises (bench presses, dips) on day one and pulling exercises (pullups, pulldowns) on day two. That way, I work different muscles."

DON'T ASSUME YOUR WORKOUTS ARE A LICENSE TO EAT. "You have to cut calories somewhere, even if you exercise. . . . You have to make a plan to sacrifice foods from somewhere in your diet."

Part 2
Busting Your Belly

Diet Theories
and Actualities

YOU PROBABLY HAVE A PRETTY GOOD IDEA OF HOW YOUR PERSONAL eating habits have added some unwanted pounds. Most guys who are ready to lose weight know how they got to this point, as evidenced in our "Belly-Off Success Story" profiles.

The bigger questions are, why so many Americans are getting fatter, why it's happening now, and why it's happening so quickly. There are three common theories that attempt to answer these questions.

1. Overweight people are lazy gluttons. This theory is propagated mostly by thin people. The idea is simple: There's more food out there than ever before. Between 1960 and 1999 the number of daily calories available to the average American increased by 700 calories, according to the U.S. Department of Agriculture. And compared to 100 years ago, daily physical activity has declined by an estimated 400 calories.

More food plus less activity equals fatter people.

That seems logical. However, it's refuted by the USDA report that, despite the number of calories *available* to Americans, the number of calories men actually *consume* declined by almost 200 per day between 1965 and 1996. Yes, guys are moving less—but they're also eating less. So much for the glutton theory.

2. Overweight people are victims of evolutionary success. Let's say the primary biological imperative of any organism is to live long enough to produce the next generation, and well enough to ensure that the subsequent generation thrives. The human species spent about 500,000 years evolving into an organism with multiple strategies for survival. One of the most valuable was our ability to store nearly endless amounts of food on our bodies: There were no side-by-side refrigerator-freezers in the Paleolithic period, so we needed our potbellies to pull us through famines and other disasters.

With the invention of agriculture about 10,000 years ago, we reached the evolutionary endgame: We learned to manipulate our environment so that each generation was practically guaranteed survival.

The next 10,000 years—from the first crops to irradiated tomatoes—are just a blip in evolutionary time. Our bodies need more time to adjust to permanent abundance. They're still designed to store food like a Kenmore.

Though this is certainly a more thoughtful and generous theory than the first, it, too, suffers a major problem: The big leap in obesity in North America—which has been mirrored worldwide, even in places we think of as too poor to have the luxury of overeating—has taken place mostly in the past 20 years.

If a species can't evolve much in 10,000 years, what could possibly have happened in just 2 decades?

That brings us to the third—and, in our view, most credible—theory of modern obesity.

3. People have been fruc'd over. We already mentioned that since 1960, the average American has had an extra 700 calories' worth of food available to eat each day. Similarly, from 1970 to 1997 the availability of corn sweeteners—mostly high-fructose corn syrup—increased about 400 percent, to 615 calories per day per person. So of those 700 bonus calories per day we could consume, it's likely many of them come from a sweetener found in Mountain Dew, Snapple, and those ubiquitous cereal bars parents shove into their kids all day long.

If calories from fructose were no different than calories from any other source, we wouldn't raise an alarm. But they seem to be different, in a very bad way.

Let's say you eat a sweet snack that contains both fat and sugar, such as a candy bar. Your body produces an immediate spike of the hormones insulin and leptin. These hormones, in tandem, send a signal to your brain that you've satisfied your appetite.

If you consume snacks or beverages that are high in fructose, your body doesn't produce as much insulin and leptin, according to preliminary research at the University of California, Davis. For some reason, these foods are invisible to your body. Theoretically, you can drink three Mountain Dews, taking in almost 500 calories, and your body won't notice you've taken in any calories at all.

Another curious interloper in the American diet is refined flour. In 1997, Americans ate an average of 200 pounds of grain and cereal products per person, according to the USDA, up from 136 pounds in 1970 and 145 pounds in 1980.

Volume, though, is only part of the story, because the average '97 intake was still just two-thirds of the 300 pounds of grains Americans ate in 1909. The other factor is the type of grains we eat today. We average only one daily serving—or fewer—of whole grains. The other grains we eat have been processed, or refined, to make them more palatable and easier to digest. Refined grains such as white bread, low-fiber cereal, and white rice cause blood sugar to spike faster than it does when you eat unrefined products such as whole-wheat bread. Give your body enough blood-sugar spikes over enough months and years, and you've got a pretty good recipe for weight gain, fat gain, insulin resistance, and all the nastiness described in the previous chapters.

Here's where it gets really, really interesting—diabolical, even. Since the '70s, Americans have been introduced to a wide variety of low-fat pastries and cereal-based snack foods that are made with not only refined flour but also high-fructose corn syrup. If you've ever wondered why you can't stop eating those football-size nonfat Entenmann's pastries until you've licked the container clean, now you know.

THE AMERICAN PARADOX

You'll notice one theory that didn't make the list: Fat makes you fat. Put less fat in you, have less fat on you.

This is perhaps the least credible explanation for why the population has gotten so much fatter, for a simple reason: Fat comprises a smaller proportion of our diets than it has in recent history, yet we're still getting fatter at a dramatic pace. Researchers call it the American Paradox. We call it a bad guess turned into a national policy, with physiologically disastrous consequences.

In 1965, the average American adult ate a diet consisting of 45 percent fat. American men ages 19 to 50 ate an average of 139 grams of fat per day. Since a high-fat diet increases cholesterol, and since cholesterol had been linked to heart disease, and since heart disease was the number one killer of Americans, our medical and nutrition establishments connected the dots and hung the blame for heart disease on dietary fat.

The nation heard the message, and by 1995, fat comprised just 34 percent of the calories in the average American's daily diet. Among men ages 19 to 50, fat consumption fell to about 101 grams a day, a decrease of 27 percent.

Meanwhile, the rate of obesity among American men grew from 10.4

to 19.9 percent. The same phenomenon occurred elsewhere. In England, for example, a steady decline in fat consumption accompanied a startling rise in fatness. Between 1980 and 1991, the number of obese Brits increased 200 percent.

If any one study truly nails the difference in your body's reaction to a low-fat versus high-fat diet, it's this one from the October 2001 issue of *International Journal of Obesity*: Researchers at Boston's Brigham and Women's Hospital and Harvard Medical School put 101 overweight people on either a low-fat diet (fat was 20 percent of total calories) or a moderate-fat diet (35 percent of calories) and followed them for 18 months.

Both groups lost weight at first, but after a year and a half, the moderate-fat group had lost an average of 9 pounds per person, whereas the low-fat dieters had *gained* 6½ pounds. That difference is startling, but there

is a caveat: After 18 months, 54 percent of the moderate-fat group were still following their diet, versus only 20 percent of the low-fat participants.

Of course, that high dropout rate is a pretty resounding vote of no-confidence in the low-fat diet. Whether it works or not, this or any other diet is useless if people can't or won't stick with it.

WHEN WE GET THE URGE

There seems to be a pretty good reason why people have so much trouble with low-fat diets: Our bodies must need a certain amount of fat. This notion arises from the extensive research that's been done on food cravings.

▶ Cravings are most likely to occur around 4:00 P.M., possibly because we don't eat enough at breakfast and lunch, so our bodies tell us to eat to prevent starvation.

▶ Men tend to crave steaks and other foods rich in fat and protein, while women usually hanker for sweets. Some researchers think this is a testosterone-driven phenomenon. Since men's bodies need fat to make testosterone, and since protein helps us build muscle and prevent it from breaking down, we crave foods rich in both when we haven't eaten enough to sustain ourselves.

▶ One survey of 562 people found that men tend to crave fattier foods when they feel sexual urges, but we

Belly Busters

▶▶▶"I always ate healthy but was sold on the low-fat thing. I realized that despite the fact that I was eating very little fat, I was carbo-loading to the tune of 3,000 to 4,000 calories a day. I switched to a more balanced diet. . . . I cut out the pasta, potatoes, cookies, juices, and soda; and stuck more to fruits, vegetables, lean meat, and fish. I drank only water and skim milk."◀◀

—CHRIS SLABON
33, LOST 40 POUNDS

don't desire high-fat foods after sex. Women, conversely, have a greater desire for fatty foods after sex. The explanation seems twofold: Before sex, you want testosterone-boosting food. (After sex, you just want sleep.) Your woman wants fattier food after sex in case her body needs to start sustaining an embryo.

THE PROS OF PROTEIN

Fat isn't the only maligned nutrient in the American diet. Protein has also taken its share of potshots. Nutritionists are quick to tell you that some minimal number like 50 grams a day or 12 to 15 percent of total calories is just fine for anyone. And they're absolutely correct—if all you want to do is survive from one year to the next. If you'd rather lose weight without losing muscle, you have to ignore them and get more protein in your diet.

One of the best examples of why a higher-protein diet works comes from a 1999 study, also published in the *International Journal of Obesity*. In it, Danish researchers put 65 subjects on either a 12-percent-protein diet, a 25-percent-protein diet, or no diet (the control group). In the first two groups, 30 percent of calories came from fat.

Unlike in the study mentioned earlier, more than 90 percent of the subjects in the Danish study completed the 6-month trial. And the results bordered on astounding.

The low-protein dieters lost more than an average of 11 pounds, which isn't bad. The high-protein subjects,

Belly Busters

▶▶"My diet for my entire life had been almost entirely carbohydrates. For example, at breakfast, I would eat nothing but cereals or breads. At dinner, I would eat an entire meal of pasta or some other carb.

"Realizing what I was doing to myself, I began to ensure that I always ate a protein at every meal with a carb. The amount of each carb would not be greater than the amount of protein. This to me was a formula that was—and still is—very easy to follow."◀◀

—DARYN HOBAL
31, LOST 30 POUNDS

however, lost an average of 20 pounds. On top of that, those in the high-protein group lost twice as much abdominal fat.

The researchers noted that both groups of dieters were highly motivated to succeed. (Unlike the 15 poor schlubs in the control group, who ate whatever they wanted and gained weight and put on almost as much abdominal fat as the low-protein group lost.) The dieters in the high-protein group nevertheless ended up eating fewer calories per day than the low-protein group.

Credit this decrease in appetite to the well-known satiating effect of protein. Protein makes you feel fuller faster, as if you've eaten a satisfying meal. Some carbohydrates can have this effect. For example, potatoes and other starches have been shown to sat-

Belly Busters

▶▶"I decided to save money and quit eating out all week. I changed my eating out to Friday and Saturday nights only. This not only saved money but allowed me to eat better—and less—at home. And it was a good thing I was saving food money, because I had to replace my clothes every 3 months."◀◀

—KEVIN SEBESTA
31, LOST 140 POUNDS

isfy your appetite faster than other foods. The effect of starches is transitory, though. You digest them quickly and then get hungry again. Fiber slows down digestion, so if you eat whole-grain bread, you should get a protein-like effect on your overall appetite. But in the Danish study, dieters in the low-protein group got more fiber than those in the high-protein group. So while fiber can reduce appetite, protein seems to do it better.

Before you move on to the next chapter—which includes a closer look at some popular diets, and why they might or might not work for you—we ask you to make sure you've digested two important pieces of information:

1. Your body seems to have a natural preference for a certain level of dietary fat. When you eat less fat early in the day, you tend to crave it later in the day. It's impossible to say what any one person's ideal dietary-fat percentage is; it probably fluctuates from day to day. (One study, for example, showed that men crave more fat after a high-intensity workout.) It seems safe to say that since some people have trouble sticking with a diet that's 20 percent fat, adherence becomes easier with a higher-fat diet—say, between 30 and 35 percent fat. This indicates that the higher percentage is a more natural level for most of us.

2. Protein helps you eat less. Even if you eat plenty of fat and steadily lose weight on a low-protein diet, you'd do even better if you ate more protein. The Danish study cited in this chapter demonstrated this phenomenon with the greater weight loss on the 25 percent protein diet. That may or may not be a magic number—we don't know whether you'd get the same results with 20 percent or 30 percent protein—but we do know 25 percent works.

He's Playing a New Tune

LIFE IN THE FAT LANE

Trumpet players have a reputation for being wild men. So Rey Sifuentes Jr., a trumpeter who marched with the Texas A&M University–Kingsville band, did his best to uphold the tradition: When he stepped into a restaurant, it was demolition time.

"I was the ultimate all-you-can-eat-buffet slayer," he says. "I'd walk into a buffet, and I could just see the managers looking at me like, 'Oh, dude, we're going to take a hit here.' "

Sifuentes routinely made four or five trips through the buffet, piling his plate high with fried chicken, french fries, and other greasy foods. "I was just an eating machine, and the stuff I was wolfing down was never anything healthy," he says. "Eating seven pieces of fried chicken was no problem for me—and even that did not satisfy the bottomless pit that was my stomach."

Eventually, however, Sifuentes's appetite for destruction caught up with him. He couldn't see his feet. He couldn't squeeze into chairs with armrests.

He didn't even have enough wind to give his trumpet a good blast.

At age 26, Sifuentes weighed 317 pounds, wore size-52 pants, and woke up every morning to the jiggle of his quadruple chins.

THE TURNING POINT

During the summer of 2000, Sifuentes took a hard look in the mirror.

"Only half of me fit," he says.

He realized he had been medicating himself with food. He ate because he was angry about losing a job, sad about not getting a new job, or bored. Often, he ate when he wasn't even hungry. "It was a quick fix for me," he says.

As he gazed at his equator-size waistline, he knew there had to be a better way to cope with stress. "I said to myself, 'You know what, dude? You need to do something about this.' "

THE PLAN OF ATTACK

Sifuentes had at times lost up to 40 pounds, only to lose motivation, stop exercising, and gain it all back. This time, he was determined to make a permanent change.

To stifle his food cravings, Sifuentes started drinking an ocean of water: a minimum of 150 ounces daily.

He began cooking healthier foods at home. Instead of eating two or three huge meals, he ate four or five smaller meals spread throughout the day. His diet included lots of baked chicken,

(continued)

Name: REY SIFUENTES JR.
Date of Birth: January 1974
Residence: San Antonio
Occupation: Reporter/sportswriter
Height: 5 foot 10

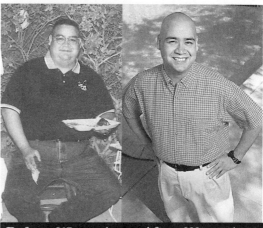

Before: 317 pounds   **After:** 226 pounds

and white rice mixed with corn. If he wanted french fries, he baked them.

For exercise, Sifuentes went to a nearby running track. "I put on my Walkman, listened to fast-paced music, and started walking," he says. After reaching the point where he could walk 5 miles, he started jogging.

Inside his apartment, he developed an all-you-can-eat exercise program that included tae kwon do, Tae Bo, aerobics, weight lifting, and shadow-boxing.

When the weather permitted, Sifuentes went outside with a football and threw bullet passes at a laundry basket wrapped with duct tape.

"Sometimes you have to do what you don't enjoy, like jogging, because it has proven benefits," he says. "But you also need to do something that you do enjoy. That way, you're more likely to stick with the workout."

In 4 months, Sifuentes lost 30 pounds. By the summer of 2001, he had lost 90 pounds.

"I have gone from wearing a size-52 pants to a size 40, which rocks," he says.

LIFE IN THE FIT LANE

Although Sifuentes still considers himself a work in progress, he's delighted with his new size.

He can see his feet and sit in any chair.

His once-monstrous appetite is now under control. "I can no longer eat as much food in one sitting," he says. "I can actually tell myself, 'Hey, dude, I'm not hungry anymore, so we can stop eating now.'"

With nearly 100 fewer pounds of himself to feed, he bounds up stairways that once exhausted him after a single flight. "I have more energy," he says. "I'm not tired all the time, the way I used to be."

As for his music, he's once again hitting those high Cs. "It has helped my trumpet playing," he says. "I'm able to use my diaphragm better."

He hasn't totally given up his old ways. A couple of times a month, he treats himself to a Wendy's triple hamburger or a trip to the all-you-can-eat buffet. "I'm still a big eater," he says. "I'm not going tell you that I only eat brussels sprouts and rice cakes. But the greasy foods, the snacks, all the stuff that tastes good and is bad for you, used to be my core diet. It's not anymore."

"I still have a bit of a tummy. I'm not magazine-cover material yet. But I just want to keep at it and see how much more I can lose. Hopefully, 40 or 50 more pounds."

HIS TIPS

DON'T EXPECT INSTANT RE-SULTS. "When you first start out, it seems kind of hopeless because, as they say, the road of 1,000 miles begins with a single step. You're not going to see results for a while."

ALWAYS RAISE THE BENCH-MARK. "You have to start small. I would walk 1 mile one day; then the next day, I'd add an extra lap at the track."

NO EXCUSES. "The next time you feel like skipping a workout, just remember what it feels like when people in public snicker at the fat-and-jolly you."

KEEP A MEMENTO. "I still have the belt that I wore when I was a size 52. It shows how far I've come and serves as a reminder of where I could end up again."

Do Diets Work?

NINETY-FIVE PERCENT OF DIETERS REGAIN ALL THEIR WEIGHT."
You've heard this one before—probably a bunch of times, since it seems to have been accepted as fact sometime back in the 1950s. Still, more than 50 years later, no one knows if this "fact" is really true. Researchers now believe it would be impossible for anyone to calculate a reliable national weight-regain statistic.

That's because, at any given time, 15 to 35 percent of Americans are on some kind of weight-loss quest, spending $33 billion a year on weight-loss products and services. There's no representative sample to test, because people try to lose weight so many ways and have such unpredictable starts and finishes. Any study would end up comparing apples to oranges.

Even if you could get a group of people to start the exact same diet on the exact same day, there'd be multiple ways to interpret the results.

Let's say three guys all start the North Hollywood Diet on the same day. (The NHD is like the Beverly Hills and Scarsdale Diets, only down-market.) All three lose weight initially. Two years later, one of them is 25 pounds lighter than before the diet, one is the same weight as before, and one is 25 pounds

Belly Busters

▶▶ "My strategy was simple: I didn't eat anything that was fattening, fried, fast food, or just plain not good for me."◀◀

—JOEY CALLAWAY
26, LOST 185 POUNDS

heavier. How do you describe those results?

You could say the diet has no benefit, since the first and third guys cancel each other out. Or, if you're trying to market *The North Hollywood Diet* on Amazon.com, you could say that 33 percent of people who try it lose 25 pounds.

What do you make of the guy who ended up back at his pre-diet weight? You'd spin that to show that he came out ahead, since he probably would've gained a pound or two if he hadn't been on the NHD. So two-thirds of people who try this diet get long-term results, and the author gets a 3-minute spot on *Good Morning America*.

However, the author of *The Sherman Oaks Diet* interprets the NHD

Belly Busters

▶▶ "Basically, my diet consists of vegetables, raw and steamed; and a lot of seafood, especially tuna for protein. I eat as many vegetables as I want and never feel hungry."◀◀

—FRANK SERAFINI
30, LOST 80 POUNDS

results differently. Since the second and third guys did lose weight initially, he calls a reporter for the *Los Angeles Times* and declares that the rival North Hollywood Diet is a colossal failure: Two-thirds of the people who try it regain all the weight they've lost. One-third of them suffer a rebound effect that causes them to gain 25 pounds.

In other words, the North Hollywood Diet doesn't reverse or prevent obesity, it causes it!

When this story breaks, someone somewhere notes that 95 percent of all dieters regain the weight they lost. Meanwhile, Krispy Kreme sales remain strong, and Dr. Atkins sells another half-million books.

LOSING WEIGHT OR LOSING HOPE?

Of course, if the author of *The North Hollywood Diet* actually had 2 years' worth of data to support or debunk his program, he'd be unique in the world of fad diets. We really know next to nothing about which diets work and which fail in the long run, despite the fact that we all know someone who's lost weight and kept it off. Something must work; we just don't have much long-term scientific data to tell us just what it is.

That's why the National Weight Control Registry, founded in 1994, gets so much attention. Its 3,500-plus members have lost at least 30 pounds and kept off the weight for at least a year, providing tons of data to the researchers who founded it. In theory, this data should point us toward the true path to permanent weight control.

The registry's members are mostly female (78 percent). They perform an admirable volume of exercise, expending approximately 2,817 calories a week through physical activity. Let's put that in perspective: To burn that many calories in a week, a 180-pound man who runs for exercise would have to cover 21½ miles. That's equal to 4 hours a week at a 5-mph pace.

As for diet, registry members are most likely to have gone the low-fat, high-carbohydrate route, with daily intakes of about 24 percent fat and about 200 grams of carbs. A recent survey showed that just 7.6 percent of the members followed high-fat, low-carbohydrate diets, such as the one advocated in *Dr. Atkins' New Diet Revolution*. Worse, those low-carb dieters maintained their weight loss for less time and performed less exercise, on average, than other registry members.

So it would appear that the case is closed: Low-fat, high-carb diets are the only way to lose a lot of weight and keep it off.

Except for this: The researchers who founded the registry recently compared a conventional low-fat diet to the Atkins diet in a 12-week study— and the Atkins diet kicked ass.

Below are the stats.

This was a short-term study, so it gives us immediate results but leaves us hungry for some long-term data. Despite the fact that Dr. Robert C. Atkins has been selling books since 1972, he has yet to produce a long-term study of results from or adherence to his diet.

That said, there are some conclusions one can draw about the major categories of diets, which follow.

EXTREME LOW-FAT, HIGH-CARB DIETS

Examples: *Dr. Dean Ornish's Program for Reversing Heart Disease* and *Eat More, Weigh Less* by Dean Ornish, M.D.; *The Pritikin Permanent Weight-Loss Manual* by Nathan Pritikin, M.D.; *The Pritikin Program for Diet and Exercise* by Nathan Pritikin, M.D., and Patrick M. McGrady Jr., M.D.

The program: Fat is less than 20 percent of total calories, sometimes less than 10 percent. Protein provides 10 to 15 percent of calories, in the form of lean meat, egg whites, and fat-free dairy or soy products. (Dr. Ornish's program is vegetarian.) Sixty-five to 70 percent of calories come from carbohydrates: vegetables, fruits, whole grains, and beans, with small amounts of sugar and white flour.

(continued on page 64)

	Subjects	Subjects Who Dropped Out	Avg Wt Loss	LDL Cholesterol	HDL Cholesterol	Triglycerides
Low-Fat Diet	21	7	7.3 lb	-14.6%	-1.8%	-2.3%
Atkins Diet	21	2	18.6 lb	+8.8%	+9.8%	-19%

You Wet Your Life

You'll notice a common trait among the guys featured in the "Belly-Off Success Story" profiles: Almost all drink more than a gallon of water a day. Here are the most common questions guys have about water, and the best answers we could come up with.

"Do I really need to drink eight 8-ounce glasses of water a day to stay healthy?"

That's 2 quarts a day, and to tell you the truth, it may not be enough. The National Research Council recommends a quart of water for every 1,000 calories expended. An average 200-pound guy who's moderately active probably uses about 2,800 calories a day, so 3 quarts of fluids daily should probably be the rule for men.

A Harvard study found that for every 8 ounces you drink, you lower your risk of bladder cancer by 7 percent. Drink 3 quarts, and reduce your risk by 49 percent.

Those 3 quarts don't have to be pure H_2O to count. You get 3 to 4 cups of fluid from your diet, assuming you eat close to 3,000 calories a day, says *Volumetrics* author Barbara Rolls, Ph.D., a nutrition professor at Pennsylvania State University. With the milk, soda, and juice an average guy drinks each day, an extra 6 cups a day may be all you need to get you to 3 quarts.

You do need more on days you exercise. Add an extra 8 ounces for an hour of weight lifting, 16 to 22 ounces for a 5-mile run, and 24 ounces for 45 minutes of full-court hoops.

"I've read that caffeine dehydrates me. Do I need extra water if I drink coffee or Mountain Dew?"

It doesn't, and you don't. In a study in the *Journal of the American College of Nutrition*, men who drank caffeinated beverages were as well-hydrated as guys who chugged equal amounts of water.

If you don't drink caffeine regularly, you experience a mild diuretic effect when you do partake. But it's a myth that the coffee goes straight through you and takes extra fluid with it. A cup of coffee counts as ⅔ cup of water.

Regular caffeine drinkers don't have to worry about extra water loss from those beverages. Your body has built up a tolerance to the diuretic effect, so a cup of coffee or Diet Coke pretty much equals a cup of water.

"Will drinking water help me lose weight?"

By itself, no. The theory behind that weight-loss strategy is that having water in your stomach all the time blunts your hunger. But Rolls thinks excess fluid intake may have the opposite effect: The more you drink, the more you dilute your body's electrolytes, including sodium and potassium. That means you need more food to restore electrolyte balances. A study on laboratory rats actually demonstrated this: The more the rats drank, the more they ate to restore their electrolytes.

Rolls' own research showed that foods prepared with water are more likely to stave off hunger than are "dry" foods paired with a drink. In one study, Rolls fed subjects three different meals: (1) chicken-and-rice soup made with 10 ounces of water; (2) chicken-and-rice casserole made without water; and (3) the same chicken-and-rice casserole washed down with a 10-ounce glass of water. After having the soup, the subjects ate less in a subsequent meal than they did after the other two meals.

Other than soup, the wettest foods are fruits and vegetables, with 80 to 95 percent water. Meats have 45 to 65 percent water; nuts have 2 to 5 percent.

Water by itself does have one genuine weight-loss benefit: If you drink water instead of soda, juices, and sweetened teas, you take in fewer calories.

"When I feel hungry, is it possible that I'm really just thirsty?"

Probably not, Rolls says. Look at this way: Could our species have survived if we couldn't tell the difference between thirst and hunger? It's possible to confuse the two if you're hungry and thirsty at the same time. But there's no evidence that you'll overeat just because you're thirsty.

"When I'm working out, should I have sports drinks instead of water?"

When you sweat heavily, you certainly lose electrolytes. Electrolyte replacement was the original selling point for Gatorade and other sports drinks. However, water works perfectly well for most exercisers. You can get the electrolytes back through food later in the day. There's no need to replace them as soon as you lose them.

A basic guideline: Drink 4 to 8 ounces of water after every 15 minutes of exercise. Drink more if it's an unusually hot, humid day or if you're working out harder and longer than you're used to. In the latter case, sports drinks may be useful to you. They taste better than water, so you're likely to drink more of them. For a routine workout in a climate-controlled gym, water is the clear choice.

"Is it true that by the time I feel thirsty, I'm already dehydrated?"

Sure, it's possible, especially if you're in the middle of a long run or an intense afternoon of pickup hoops. In those cases, it makes sense to anticipate thirst, rather than wait for it, Rolls says. The rest of the time, drink when you're thirsty.

Even if you're not parched, your tank is probably low if your pee is dark yellow: It should be pale and odorless. And if you notice that you don't have to whiz as often as usual or that your stream has slowed to a trickle, you probably need a fluid refill.

The theory: The diets were devised to reverse or prevent heart disease, based on the assumption that saturated fat is the primary cause of the ailment. The diets were later repositioned to capitalize on Americans' growing interest in weight loss.

The claims: Advocates claim these diets combat heart disease, diabetes type 2, high blood pressure, cancer, arthritis, stress, and the harmful effects of smoking. Dr. Pritikin also asserts that medications for heart disease, diabetes, and high blood pressure can be reduced or eliminated if you follow his diet.

Why they might work:

▶ Overweight people who go on these diets lose weight and body fat. When 2,643 men consumed a very-low-fat, high-fiber diet during a medically supervised study that also included daily aerobic exercise, each lost an average of 5.5 percent of his body weight in 3 weeks.

▶ Both the Ornish and Pritikin diets reduce total and LDL ("bad") cholesterol.

▶ Low-fat diets usually result in decreased blood-glucose and insulin levels.

▶ Some experts say very-low-fat, high-carbohydrate diets are the only ones proven to reverse atherosclerosis and decrease insulin resistance.

Why they might not be worth the trouble:

▶ These are prototypal carrot-stick diets, and adherence is notoriously low. Studies show that even some cardiac patients have trouble complying, even though it's safe to assume they've been told their lives are at stake. In other words, most guys would rather die than live on sprouts and brown rice.

▶ While low-fat diets reduce LDL cholesterol, they also cause a dip in HDL—the good stuff.

MAINSTREAM MODERATE-FAT, LOW-CALORIE DIETS

Examples: Diets based on the USDA Food Guide Pyramid, the National Cholesterol Education Program Step I and Step II Diets, and diets offered by some commercial weight-loss programs (Weight Watchers, Jenny Craig, Nutri/System).

The program: Usually 20 to 30 percent fat, 15 to 20 percent protein, and 55 to 60 percent carbohydrates. To

Belly Busters

▶▶ "Find a nutritious meal that you like and stick to it—routine is good for creating good habits. My magic meal? One chicken breast with steamed rice and vegetables and skim milk (with chocolate syrup)." ◀◀

—GEOFFREY WHITE
26, LOST MORE THAN 150 POUNDS

encourage compliance, dieters are given a wide range of food choices. The goal is a slow but steady weight loss of a pound or two a week.

The theory: No big idea here: Caloric restriction results in weight loss, and safe, steady, permanent weight loss is achieved by cutting 500 to 1,000 calories from your daily diet. The lowest recommended daily intake for men is 1,200 to 1,400 calories, or less than half of a Thanksgiving dinner.

The claims: They're safe and they work, with almost no downsides.

Why they might work:

▶ A number of studies have shown that cutting fat to below 30 percent of total calories results in significant weight loss.

▶ Health benefits include lower LDL cholesterol, lower fasting insulin levels, improved blood pressure, and, if you stay on the diets long enough, a permanent aversion to the taste of fat-rich foods.

Why they might not be worth the trouble:

▶ You can lose weight through calorie restriction even without cutting fat. For example, researchers at Castleview Hospital in Price, Utah, placed four groups of obese people on 1,200-calorie diets containing 15 percent, 20 percent, 28 percent, or 34 percent fat. Everyone lost weight and body fat, with no significant differ-

Belly Busters

▶▶▶"Step one was to start at the root of the problem and banish temptation. Out went potato chips, ice cream, cream cheese, bread, beer, butter, and hamburger. I knew if the food wasn't in my house, I couldn't eat it.

"Step two was replacing that food with healthier choices. I added more fruits and vegetables, reduced portions, and seriously monitored my fat intake. I read labels. Sweets and pastries were out. Booze was out. Fried foods—out!"◀◀

—MARK OHLINGER
31, LOST 60 POUNDS

ences in how much weight each group lost or how quickly they lost it.

▶ The diets cause reduced HDL cholesterol.

EXTREME HIGH-FAT, LOW-CARB DIETS

Examples: *Dr. Atkins' Diet Revolution* (1972; updated 20 years later as *Dr. Atkins' New Diet Revolution*) by Robert C. Atkins, M.D.; *Protein Power* by Michael R. Eades, M.D., and Mary Dan Eades, M.D.; *The Carbohydrate Addict's Diet* by Dr. Rachael F. Heller and Dr. Richard F. Heller

The program: Typically 55 to 65 percent fat, with fewer than 100 daily grams of carbohydrates and the rest protein. During the 2-week "induction" phase of the Atkins diet, for example, you can eat as much meat,

Belly Busters

▶▶"I love my grill, and it's amazing what you can do with a piece of fish and the right seasonings."◀◀

—JAMES GORDON
44, LOST 60 POUNDS

butter, cream, and eggs as you want as long as you restrict daily carbohydrate consumption to 20 grams or less—about the amount in a hot dog bun. (You consume most of the carbs in nutrient-dense mixed-green salads.) After the induction phase, you eat anywhere from 15 to 60 grams of carbs a day, the magic number for each person being that at which he stops losing weight. Carbs are later upped again, to a range of 25 to 90 daily grams.

The theory: Severe carbohydrate restriction forces the body into a state called ketosis, in which fat is readily mobilized as the primary source of fuel. Ketosis suppresses appetite and lowers blood-sugar and insulin levels, resulting in weight loss and fat loss, while preserving muscle.

The claims: Caloric intake, per se, doesn't matter in weight control. If you restrict highly addictive carbohydrates, you either lose or maintain weight—you can't possibly gain.

Why they might work:
▶ We already mentioned one recent study that showed that low-

carbohydrate diets work better than low-fat diets for weight loss. Other studies have shown positive results in overweight people who self-select such diets. Early in the diet, you lose "water weight." Carbohydrates cause your body to hold water, so when you cut carbs, you lose the water you've been holding. Over longer periods, however, low-carbohydrate diets do result in loss of body fat.

▶ People who lose weight on high-fat, low-carbohydrate diets may experience decreases in blood pressure, blood sugar, insulin levels, and triglycerides.

Why they might not be worth the trouble:
▶ No one knows the long-term effects of ketogenic diets, and you won't find many scientists who believe ketosis is necessary for weight loss.

▶ You have to take a lot of vitamin supplements to make up for the nutrients you would otherwise get through carbohydrate sources.

▶ Increases in total and LDL cholesterol can be dramatic on the Atkins diet. Some scientists calculate that long-term use of the Atkins diet increases total cholesterol by 25 percent. (However, one study found that although LDL increased on an Atkins-like diet, so did the size of the LDL particles. Small, dense LDL particles are considered dangerous, while larger, fluffier molecules are thought to be harmless.)

▶ Limiting carbohydrates may hurt your workouts; it could be tough to work out with depleted glycogen stores. If you lift weights, you may miss out on some muscle-building benefits if you don't consume any carbohydrates after your workout.

▶ In a world filled with carbohydrates, it's hard to just say no.

BALANCED-MACRONUTRIENT DIET

If you saw it on your plate, you might consider it "everything in moderation." If a nutritionist saw it, she'd probably declare it to be high in fat, high in protein, and low to moderate in carbohydrates.

We think it's the most natural, satisfying, and healthy diet for men, and in the next chapter, we'll show you how to follow it.

Active-Duty Weight Loss

LIFE IN THE FAT LANE

As the son of a career military non-commissioned officer, Lakin Lankford didn't get to put down many roots when he was growing up. Somehow, he still became as big as a prize pumpkin. "I was what I called big boned, what my parents called a big teddy bear, and what everyone else called a fat ass," he says.

Even at 250 pounds, Lankford was light enough on his feet to letter in high school tennis. "I wanted to become the heaviest player in history to play Wimbledon."

Instead of entering the professional tennis circuit, however, he entered college, where his favorite courses were breakfast, lunch, and dinner. "The cafeteria was all-you-can-eat," he says. "So I was just eating all the time."

To start his day, he ate three bowls of cereal with whole milk, followed by two breakfast sandwiches with sausage and cheese, and a stack of pan-cakes. For lunch, he ate two cheeseburgers, chili cheese fries, soda, and ice cream.

Dinner was his "healthy" meal . . . in theory. Invariably, the chicken-breast sandwich he intended to eat would turn into two sandwiches with full-fat mayonnaise. Each Wednesday, he went out with a buddy for burgers and shakes.

Lankford was so out of shape that he wouldn't walk the two uphill blocks that separated his dorm from the library. "To avoid any physical exertion, I drove my car," he says.

While others gained the freshman 15, Lankford added the freshman 40. "I put on weight like I never had before," he says. "One day, I stepped on a scale and it said 296."

His dreams of playing on the professional tennis circuit were gone. At the rate he was going, he'd soon be a candidate for the pro sumo circuit.

THE TURNING POINT

At year's end, Lankford went home with no intention of returning to school. He surprised his parents by announcing that he wanted to join the Air Force. They didn't believe me," he says. "I was weak and out of shape, big time."

With his weight, he didn't qualify for enlistment—not even close. "The maximum weight for my height was 220 pounds," he says. "I had to get under the maximum to even be processed into the military, and I had to keep it off until I went in."

Name: LAKIN LANKFORD
Date of Birth: September 1979
Residence: Arlington, Texas
Occupation: Senior Airman, U.S. Air Force
Height: 6 foot 3

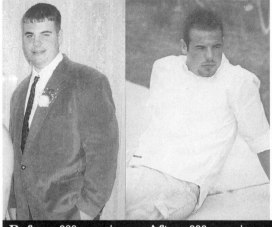

Before: 296 pounds   **After:** 220 pounds

THE PLAN OF ATTACK

That summer, Lankford worked with a surveying crew. He enjoyed being outdoors, and he listened intently as his boss extolled the virtues of a high-protein, low-carbohydrate diet.

"He got me hooked," Lankford says. "I cut out all carbohydrates, sodas, and sugar. I loaded up on steak, poultry, and fish." He could still eat bacon and eggs for breakfast, tuna with mayonnaise for lunch, and steak for dinner.

"My favorite part was I went on the diet for 12 days and then off it for 2 days," he says. "It gave me something to look forward to every 2 weeks."

He was on his feet for 9 to 10 hours a day, drank as much water as he could, and lost weight quickly—80 pounds in 4 months—despite the fact that he had no formal exercise program.

In November 1998, he signed his enlistment papers and followed his father into military service.

LIFE IN THE FIT LANE

Lankford quickly realized he wasn't exactly in fighting trim. "I was surprised by how weak I was," he says.

Basic training toughened him up. In the end, he passed all the physical tests, despite eating mountains of carbohydrate-rich military chow. "They were working me so hard that all the carbs burned right off," Lankford says.

After basic, he again limited his carbohydrate consumption and loaded up on bacon, eggs, and steak. Despite a high fat intake and a weekly cheat day when he ate whatever he wanted, his cholesterol levels stayed within normal limits.

Lankford also became a regular at the base gymnasium. At first, he worked out 5 days a week, each time incorporating 30 minutes of cardiovascular exercise and 30 minutes of strength training.

Each day, he worked a different muscle group. Mondays were for his chest; Tuesdays were for biceps; Wednesdays were for legs; Thursdays were for triceps; and Fridays were for back and shoulders. "I work each muscle till I can't lift anymore, since I only work it once a week," he says. "It gives the muscles enough time to heal."

As he bulked up, he edged past his maximum allowable weight, so he was sent for a body-fat measurement. To everyone's surprise, his fat totaled just 11 percent of his body weight, a figure many pro athletes would be proud to claim. His superiors wisely decided he was fit enough to continue serving his country.

In January 2002, Lankford married a woman he first met when he was a fat, dateless freshman. His wife doesn't remember that initial meeting—she only recalls the sterling specimen she met on New Year's Eve 2000. "I looked totally different the second time she met me," Lankford says. "We kind of hit things off."

HIS TIPS

GET JUICED. Before each meal, Lankford downs a glass of grapefruit juice. "In my stomach, it works as a catalyst to break up the food. So I feel fuller quicker."

MAKE A FIST. Lankford rations his portions by hand. "I usually eat a fist-size portion of carbs, a fist-size portion of meat, and then vegetables."

GO OFF-MENU. When Lankford eats in a restaurant, he makes menu substitutions. "You do kind of figure out how to think ahead. . . . I can get the steak, and then I can substitute extra vegetables for the bread or the potato."

The Belly-Off Diet

THE THREE TYPES OF DIETS DISCUSSED IN THE PREVIOUS CHAPTER—extreme low-fat and high-carb; mainstream moderate-fat and low-calorie; and extreme high-fat and low-carb—suffer from one major drawback: They all require a steep learning curve. You have to get your tastebuds used to less fat or fewer carbohydrates, and you have to ignore most of the food in the real world in order to make the diets work.

Trainer and nutritionist Thomas Incledon, R.D., Ph.D., believes that there's a better solution. If you want to lose weight, he says, first make sure you're getting enough protein in your diet. Protein makes you feel fuller while you're eating, and helps you build muscle and speed up your metabolism.

Next, get enough fat. Fat helps you feel fuller longer between meals, slowing your appetite. It provides essential fatty acids needed for optimal health. And it also makes you feel that you're eating real food. You never feel as if you were starving in the land of plenty. This is vital because few can make deprivation a permanent way of life.

Most important, Incledon says, is that when you have enough protein and fat, your total calorie intake takes care of itself. You still need to pay attention to what you're eating at every meal. You still need to know which foods to avoid. But you don't have to starve or make a daily treadmill death march to lose weight. You just need to give your body what it needs, when it needs it, and let the food do its work, in conjunction with whatever exercise program you choose to follow.

So in developing the Belly-Off diet, our first goal was to make sure the above considerations were built in. We wanted a template you could use anywhere, anytime, with minimal calculation. And we wanted a diet that you could self-regulate by easily adding more fat and protein when you feel you need it, or subtracting some when you don't. Our aim was to ensure that there's no point in the day when you're starving or craving a jelly doughnut.

Here's how Incledon built the sample diet in this chapter.

Protein. Chapter 6 discussed a Danish study that showed a 25 percent protein diet reduces appetite and speeds weight loss. A range of protein from 20 to 30 percent of calories may have the same effect, but Incledon chose 25 percent for the sample diet.

Fat. Incledon believes that each guy has a natural fat intake that could range from 20 to 40 percent of his total calories. If you go below your natural intake, you'll probably start to crave

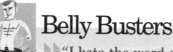

Belly Busters

▶▶ "I hate the word *diet*, so I prefer to call it *food-consumption modification*." ◀◀

— JEFFREY CHADWICK
43, LOST 80 POUNDS

high-fat foods. The sample diet features 30 percent fat, but you can easily adjust it to fit your fat preference as it changes from day to day.

Carbohydrates. These simply fill out the rest of your plate. In the sample, they're 45 percent of calories, with a lot of vegetables, fruits, and whole grains.

SEEKING THE BALANCE

The proportions of Incledon's sample diet work out to 25-30-45 (protein-fat-carbohydrate), which isn't snappy but also isn't all that important. The reason balanced-macronutrient diets seem to work better than others isn't because of some magical zone you hit when the numbers line up a particular way. It's because you eat enough protein to feel satisfied and full after any given meal, enough fat to stave off cravings later in the day, and enough carbohydrates to give your palate a full range of tastes and your body a combination of fast- and slow-burning fuel sources.

There are three keys to making a balanced-macronutrient diet work.

1. Include some of each macronutrient in each meal. Again, this is not to comply with any zoning ordinance but to ensure that (a) your body has all the nutrients it needs at every point in the day, (b) you feel full for as long as possible between meals, and (c) you minimize cravings.

2. When you're hungry, eat real food. With one exception (which we'll discuss in the next section), you should eat only food that you can picture in its natural, pre-processed state. When you see a hunk of beef, you can visualize a cow. When you see a salad, you can visualize lettuce growing out of the ground; and when you look at olive oil–based salad dressing, you can envision an olive tree on a sun-drenched hillside in Sicily.

So what do you contemplate when you look at a Twinkie or a bottle of Snapple? Can you conceive of herds of wild Snapple stampeding through an Arizona canyon? A Twinkie vine climbing up the canyon wall?

3. Anticipate your cravings, and trust your instincts. Your first defense against

Belly Busters

▶▶ "[My wife and I] haven't changed the kinds of foods we eat, but we have changed the portions and the methods of cooking. Moderation is the key.

"We eat out frequently and haven't encountered problems. There are plenty of healthy menus available. We avoid cream sauces and anything deep-fried, battered, or breaded. We opt for food that's grilled, roasted, baked, or broiled, and order dressing on the side. It works." ◀◀

—DON FITZGERALD
67, LOST 153 POUNDS

cravings, as mentioned, is regular meals and snacks, such as the ones in the sample diet that follows.

Although there's nothing simple about cravings, they are real. A craving for pizza may be your body telling you to eat fat and protein. Or it may not be—it's anyone's guess whether your body actually has this self-regulatory capability. Whatever the cause, you want to call Domino's. Same with salty or spicy foods: Your body may be telling you it needs salt or spice, or it could be saying something else altogether. A yearning for salty, sour, or spicy food could be a fat craving in disguise.

If stress prompts you to crave sweets, your brain may need more serotonin or endorphins, feel-good hormones triggered by carbohydrates.

HOW TO USE THE DIET

The meals shown are "templates" that you can vary any number of ways to please your individual tastebuds and avoid eating the same old thing every day. Detailed information about calories, protein, fat, and carbohydrates is given for each item in each meal. It's not a bad idea to photocopy the templates and carry them with you to the grocery store so you buy food that fits those parameters.

You don't have to hit the calorie counts on the nose. If, for instance, you eat a dish with more fat than shown here, simply eat less fat in your next meal.

The templates include two breakfast options: cereal and an omelet. The cereal (which can be hot or cold, Raisin

Bran or old-fashioned oatmeal) has about 100 fewer calories. The omelet is ideal right after a workout, if you exercise first thing in the morning, or the morning after an afternoon or evening workout.

There's only one lunch shown. (We know that you eat the same lunch everyday, just like we do.) Still, you can create infinite variations: different types of bread, different meat, different cheese, different condiments, different vegetables.

For dinner, choose one food item from each of the six categories in the template: meat, salad, dressing, dark green vegetable, starch, and fruit. You can riff on those variables any number of ways. (You'll find four dinner examples right after the meal templates.) Make sure the nutrient values of the foods you choose add up to 700 to 800 total calories, 44 to 50 grams of protein, 23 to 27 grams of fat, and 79 to 90 grams of carbohydrates. Staying within these ranges will ensure that you get the right mix of protein, fat, and carbs.

The nutrient values listed for meats refer to raw 5-ounce cuts; keep in mind that sauces, breading, oil, and other ingredients used during cooking will tack on additional calories, fat, and carbohydrates. The healthiest ways to prepare meats are grilling, baking, broiling, and stir-frying with a small amount of canola or olive oil. Likewise, adding butter or margarine to starches such as bread or potatoes or to vegetables will increase the nutrient values of those foods. When it comes to cooking vegetables, we recommend steaming them until they're crisp-tender.

Belly Busters

▶▶ "I started with the usual low-calorie microwavable dinners that taste like crap. I could see this wasn't going to work. So I started buying magazines such as *Men's Health* to learn more about food.

"To my amazement, there are piles of good food out there. When the food was cooked right and with the proper ingredients, the weight started coming off. I was amazed at the results." ◀◀

—JEFF SOVERAN
39, LOST 42 POUNDS

Each day, in addition to your three square meals, you should eat a "floater" fourth meal. Two of the floater-meal templates can be either eaten as a full meal or divided in half and used as two snacks—2 hours before lunch and 2 hours after, for example. A third floater template is a protein shake for workout days: You can have the entire thing after a workout, or drink half an hour before exercise and the rest immediately after.

The meal plan as written should give you between 2,400 and 2,800 calories a day. This should provide plenty of calories for all but the most severely obese, while allowing most guys to lose fat at a steady pace. (If you are severely obese, please consult your doctor before you try this diet or any other.)

A 2,800-calorie diet should allow a mostly sedentary 300-pound guy to lose about a pound a week. If you're bigger or more active, you'll lose more weight on that diet. If you're lighter or less active, you'll shed fewer pounds. For instance, a moderately active 200-pounder might get no weight reduction from

2,800 calories a day but lose a pound every other week at 2,400 calories. Each guy is different. You can't really know what calorie count you need until you try it.

The emphasis on protein should allow weight lifters to gain muscle and perhaps prevent the aerobic exercisers from losing much. Whatever your exercise program, you might find you prefer the higher-calorie options on the days you exercise. Or you might not. The whole point is to make this diet as instinctive as possible.

At Least You Don't Have to Eat Curds, Too

The protein shake, which contains whey protein and flaxseed oil, is the only part of the Belly-Off diet that violates the dictum "Eat only food that you can picture in its natural, pre-processed state." We don't know about you, but when we try to picture whey, all we get are images of Little Miss Muffet.

It turns out that whey is a milk protein, but outside of nursery rhymes, we've never seen it in any form other than a powder you buy in plastic jugs at GNC. New research has shown some compelling reasons to include whey protein in your diet. First, of course, is its muscle-building benefit. In a 2001 study in the *International Journal of Sport Nutrition and Exercise Metabolism*, experienced weight lifters gained 5 pounds of muscle in 6 weeks of supplementation with whey protein. A placebo group did the same workout routine without the protein supplements and gained just 2 pounds. Whey also has been shown to improve your immune system and have some antioxidant effects.

No research has ever compared whey protein to real food, in equal amounts and at the same times of day, to see if the supplement works better, or if real food is just as good, notes Thomas Incledon, R.D., Ph.D. But we now have evidence that supplementing your regular diet with whey protein will help you build more muscle than you would without supplementing.

Shopping for a protein powder is intimidating at first, but you get the hang of it pretty quickly. We like GNC's house brand, Mega Whey, along with NITRO-Tech from MuscleTech. Incledon recommends Nature's Best-Isopure and whey-protein powders from HDT and Proteinlab. The only way to go wrong is to buy the cheapest one in the store from a company you've never heard of; the more expensive, better-known brands tend to be superior in taste and quality. (Cheaper versions may be blends of poor-quality proteins, or contain excess lactose, making them more difficult for some people to digest.)

When preparing your whey-protein shake, mix in flaxseed oil. There's no great trick to buying flaxseed oil, but you have to remember to keep it refrigerated. It quickly goes rancid at room temperature.

MEAL TEMPLATES

Depending on how creative you are, you can go weeks without having the exact same meal, despite the fact that you get about the same number of calories each time.

BREAKFAST 1

Food	Amount	Calories	Protein (g)	Fat (g)	Carbs (g)
Cereal or oatmeal, whole grain	1¼ cup	155	4	0	33
Milk, fat-free	2 cups	170	17	1	24
Almonds or other nuts	4 Tbsp	205	7	17	7
Raisins, seedless	2 Tbsp	61	1	0	14
Total		591	29	18	78

BREAKFAST 2 (POST-WORKOUT)

Food	Amount	Calories	Protein (g)	Fat (g)	Carbs (g)
Omelet made with:		178	25	5	8
Whole egg	1				
Egg whites	5				
Peppers and onions	½ cup				
Milk, fat-free	1 cup	85	8	0	12
Bread, whole grain	2 slices	167	6	2	31
Margarine	1 Tbsp	103	0	11	0
Fruit (e.g., banana, apple, pear, orange)	1 large	116	1	1	27
Total		649	40	19	78

LUNCH

Food	Amount	Calories	Protein (g)	Fat (g)	Carbs (g)
Sandwich made with:		518	38	24	38
Lunchmeat or drained canned tuna	5 oz				
Cheese, reduced-fat	1 slice				
Romaine lettuce	2 leaves				
Tomato	2 slices				
Mayonnaise	1 Tbsp				
Bread, whole grain	2 slices				
Carrot	1	33	1	0	7
Orange juice	1 cup	115	2	1	26
Total		666	41	25	71

DINNER

Food	Amount	Calories	Protein (g)	Fat (g)	Carbs (g)
Meat:					
Pork tenderloin	5 oz raw	147	30	3	0
Chicken breast, boneless and skinless	5 oz raw	150	33	2	0
Turkey breast, boneless and skinless	5 oz raw	150	33	2	0
Turkey ham	5 oz raw	175	27	7	1
Beef, lean, such as	5 oz raw				
Round		187	31	7	0
Ground beef, 90% lean		233	29	13	0
Flank steak		247	28	15	0
Sirloin		315	27	23	0
Seafood, such as	5 oz raw				
Clams		97	18	1	4
Cod		109	25	1	0
Haddock		117	27	1	0
Flounder		126	27	2	0
Shrimp		138	29	2	1
Tuna		141	33	1	0
Halibut		147	30	3	0
Catfish		158	26	6	0
Salmon		193	28	9	0
Trout		201	30	9	0
Salad:	1 cup				
Romaine lettuce		8	1	0	1
Green leaf lettuce		12	1	0	2
Spinach		16	2	0	2
Salad dressing:	2 Tbsp				
Ranch		107	1	11	1
Thousand Island		119	0	11	5
Caesar		134	0	14	2
French		137	0	13	5
Italian		138	0	14	3
Oil and vinegar		148	0	16	1

Food	Amount	Calories	Protein (g)	Fat (g)	Carbs (g)
Dark green vegetable:	1 cup				
Green beans		48	2	0	10
Broccoli		55	5	1	8
Asparagus	about 8 spears	63	5	1	9
Snow peas		64	5	0	11
Brussels sprouts		77	4	1	14
Artichokes		89	5	1	15
Sweet peas		136	9	0	25
Starch:					
Bread (wheat, rye, or pumpernickel)	1 slice	81	3	1	15
Potato, russet or red-skin	1 medium	112	3	0	25
Sweet potato	1 medium	136	2	0	32
Pasta, whole wheat (e.g. spaghetti)	1 cup	185	7	1	37
Couscous	1 cup	196	7	0	42
Barley	1 cup	201	4	1	44
Rice, whole grain	1 cup	222	5	2	46
Fruit:					
Strawberries	¾ cup	38	1	0	8
Watermelon chunks	¾ cup	38	1	0	8
Cantaloupe chunks	¾ cup	44	1	0	10
Peach	1 medium	48	1	0	11
Grapes	¾ cup	51	1	1	12
Raspberries	¾ cup	57	1	1	11
Grapefruit	¾ cup	60	1	0	14
Pineapple chunks	¾ cup	61	0	1	14
Blueberries	¾ cup	64	1	0	15
Orange	1 medium	88	1	0	21
Apple	1 medium	90	0	1	21
Pear	1 medium	113	1	1	25
Banana	1 medium	116	1	1	27

FLOATER 1 (NON-EXERCISE DAYS)*

Food	Amount	Calories	Protein (g)	Fat (g)	Carbs (g)
Bread, whole grain	2 slices	167	6	2	31
Peanut butter	2 Tbsp	202	8	16	7
Milk, fat-free	2 cups	170	17	1	24
Apple	1 medium	90	0	1	21
Total		**629**	**31**	**20**	**83**

* Eat as one meal or two snacks

FLOATER 2 (EXERCISE OR NON-EXERCISE DAYS)**

Food	Amount	Calories	Protein (g)	Fat (g)	Carbs (g)
Cottage cheese, fat-free	1 cup	152	26	0	12
Pineapple, canned, water-packed	5 oz	81	1	0	19
Crackers, whole wheat	10	208	4	8	31
Cashews or other nuts	¼ cup	200	5	16	9
Total		**641**	**36**	**24**	**71**

** Eat as one meal or two snacks

FLOATER 3 (EXERCISE DAYS)***

Food	Amount	Calories	Protein (g)	Fat (g)	Carbs (g)
Protein shake with:					
Whey protein powder	4 Tbsp	220	35	0	20
Blueberries	1 cup	93	1	1	21
Flaxseed oil	1½ Tbsp	189	0	21	0
Orange juice	1½ cups	172	3	1	39
Total		**674**	**39**	**23**	**80**

*** Drink in its entirety as post-workout shake, or drink half 1 hour before exercise and the other half immediately after

FOUR SAMPLE DINNERS

CHICKEN DINNER

Food	Amount	Calories	Protein (g)	Fat (g)	Carbs (g)
Grilled Chicken Caesar Salad	1 serving (5 oz chicken, 3 cups salad with dressing)	516	44	25	29
Rolls, whole wheat	2	192	7	2	37
Pineapple, sliced	1 cup	85	1	1	19
Total		793	52	28	85

Skill Level: Easy

Prep and Cooking Time: You'll need about 10 minutes to grill the chicken and 10 minutes to prepare the salad, for a total of 20 minutes.

If you barbecue on Sunday, grill a few extra chicken breasts without barbecue sauce. Later in the week, use them in the Grilled Chicken Caesar Salad.

Grilled Chicken Caesar Salad

Salad

2	cups romaine lettuce, chopped
1	cup baby spinach
1	cup prepared croutons
1	5-ounce skinless chicken breast, grilled and sliced

Dressing

2	tablespoons lemon juice
1½	tablespoons olive oil
1	tablespoon Parmesan cheese
2	teaspoons mustard
1	teaspoon Worcestershire sauce
	Dash of hot-pepper sauce

To make the salad: In a medium bowl, combine the lettuce, spinach, croutons, and chicken.

To make the dressing: In a small bowl, combine the lemon juice, oil, cheese, mustard, Worcestershire sauce, and hot-pepper sauce. Toss with the salad.

Serves 1

LEAN-BEEF DINNER

Food	Amount	Calories	Protein (g)	Fat (g)	Carbs (g)
Steak and Mushrooms	1 serving (5 oz steak)	267	29	15	3
Easy Fruit Salad with Walnut Vinaigrette	1 serving (1 cup salad, ¾ cup fruit)	201	2	8	30
Asparagus, steamed	1 cup (about ½ frozen 9-oz pkg)	63	5	1	9
Near East wheat-pilaf mix, prepared according to pkg directions	1 cup	192	6	0	42
Total		723	42	24	84

Skill Level: Some measuring and chopping. You have the technology.

Prep and Cooking Time: About 20 minutes for the steak dish, about 10 minutes for the fruit salad, 5 to 7 minutes for the asparagus, and about 20 minutes for the pilaf. With a little coordination, this meal can be ready in a half-hour.

Steak and Mushrooms

1¼   pounds (20 oz) flank steak
¼   teaspoon salt
⅛   teaspoon ground black pepper
1   package (8 oz) sliced mushrooms
¼   cup water
1   teaspoon Worcestershire sauce
1   teaspoon minced garlic

Coat a medium skillet with olive oil cooking spray and heat over medium-high heat. Sprinkle the steak with the salt and pepper. Place the steak in the skillet and cook for 6 to 7 minutes. Spray the steak with the olive oil, turn, and cook for another 6 to 7 minutes for medium-rare.

Remove the steak to a plate. Cover to keep warm.

Add the remaining ingredients to the skillet. Stir to scrape up any brown bits. Cook for 5 to 6 minutes, or until the mushrooms soften. Slice the steak, and top with the prepared mushroom sauce.

Makes 4 servings

Easy Fruit Salad with Walnut Vinaigrette

Salad

- 4   cups torn bibb lettuce or fresh baby spinach leaves
- 4   kiwifruit, peeled and sliced
- 1   cup jarred mango
- ½   avocado, peeled, pitted, and diced

Vinaigrette

- 1   tablespoon honey
- 1   tablespoon canola or olive oil
- ¼   cup orange juice
- 1   tablespoon lime juice

To make the salad: Divide the lettuce among 4 salad plates. To one plate, add ¼ of the kiwi slices, ¼ cup of the mango, and ¼ of the avocado. Repeat with the remaining ingredients.

To make the dressing: In a small bowl, whisk together the honey and oil. Slowly whisk in the orange juice and lime juice. Drizzle over each of the 4 prepared salads.

Makes 4 servings

HADDOCK DINNER

Food	Amount	Calories	Protein (g)	Fat (g)	Carbs (g)
Lemon-Pepper Haddock with Jalapeños	1 serving (5-oz fish fillet)	136	27	3	1
Creole Spinach Salad with Dressing	1 serving	152	4	11	10
Goya black-beans-and-rice mix, prepared according to pkg directions	1 cup	413	10	11	68
Strawberries	¾ cup	38	1	0	8
Total		**739**	**42**	**25**	**87**

Skill Level: Just slice and mix.

Prep and Cooking Time: About 20 minutes for the fish dish. If you use pre-washed spinach (and you should), the salad should take about 5 minutes. The beans-and-rice mixture takes about 20 minutes to prepare.

Cook the rice first, prep the fish and pop it in the oven, then throw the salad together. You'll be eating in 30 minutes.

Lemon-Pepper Haddock with Jalapeños

4   5-oz firm-flesh fish fillets, such as haddock or cod
¼   cup low-fat Italian salad dressing
2   scallions, sliced
1   jalapeño pepper, seeded and chopped (wear plastic gloves when handling)
2   teaspoons lemon-pepper seasoning
¼   teaspoon salt

Preheat the oven to 375°F. Cut 4 pieces of foil, each about 10" long, depending on the size of the fillets. Place a fillet on a piece of foil. Top with 1 tablespoon of the salad dressing, ¼ of the scallions, ¼ of the jalapeño pepper, ½ teaspoon of the lemon-pepper seasoning, and a pinch of the salt. Cover with another piece of foil and crimp edges to seal. Repeat with the remaining ingredients. Place the foil packets on a baking sheet. Bake for 10 minutes, or until the fish flakes easily when tested with a fork.

Makes 4 servings

Creole Spinach Salad with Dressing

Salad
1   pound fresh spinach, washed and trimmed of tough stems
1   red onion, thinly sliced

Dressing
3   tablespoons olive oil
2   tablespoons Dijon mustard
2   tablespoons lemon juice
2   tablespoons balsamic vinegar
1   teaspoon Creole seasoning
     Hot-pepper sauce
     Ground white pepper

To make the salad: In a large bowl, toss together the spinach and red onion.

To make the dressing: In a blender, combine the oil, mustard, lemon juice, vinegar, Creole seasoning, and the hot-pepper sauce and white pepper to taste. Process on high for 1 minute. Pour over the salad. Toss well to combine.

Makes 4 servings

CATFISH DINNER

Food	Amount	Calories	Protein (g)	Fat (g)	Carbs (g)
Light Catfish Fry	1 serving (5-oz fish fillet)	229	33	8	6
Coleslaw	1 serving	183	1	14	14
Baked Sweet Potato Wedges	1 serving	159	2	3	32
Broccoli florets, steamed	1 cup	55	5	1	8
Pears, canned	¾ cup	100	1	0	24
Total		726	42	26	84

Skill Level: Have a set of measuring spoons on hand.

Prep and Cooking Time: The fish should take about 15 minutes of prep time. The potatoes can be prepped in about 5. You can bake the two together, which will take approximately 20 minutes. The broccoli should take about 15 minutes; the coleslaw only 5. You could prepare them while the fish and potatoes are baking. Total time is about 40 minutes.

Light Catfish Fry

1½ pounds catfish or haddock fillet
2 tablespoons Dijon mustard
1 tablespoon fat-free plain yogurt
1 tablespoon chopped chives
1 tablespoon chopped fresh parsley
Pinch of ground red pepper
1 cup fresh bread crumbs

Rinse the fish fillets and pat dry. Cut the fillets into a total of 8 equal pieces. In a cup, combine the mustard, yogurt, chives, parsley, and ground red pepper. Rub the mustard mixture onto all sides of each piece of fish. Place the fish on a plate, cover, and refrigerate for about 30 minutes.

Preheat the oven to 375°F. Coat a baking sheet with cooking spray. Thoroughly coat the fish pieces with the bread crumbs. Place the fish on the prepared baking sheet and bake for 10 to 12 minutes, or until the fish flakes easily when tested with a fork.

Makes 4 servings

Coleslaw

1½	cups packaged coleslaw
1	tablespoon pickle relish
1	tablespoon vinegar
1	tablespoon oil
1	teaspoon mustard
¼	teaspoon salt
	Pinch of ground black pepper

Place the coleslaw in a small bowl. In a cup, combine the relish, vinegar, oil, mustard, salt, and pepper. Pour over the coleslaw and mix well.

Makes 1 serving

Baked Sweet Potato Wedges

1	sweet potato
½	teaspoon canola or olive oil

Cut the sweet potato into 4 to 6 wedges. In a small bowl, toss the wedges with the oil. Place the wedges on the baking sheet with the Light Catfish Fry and bake in the 375°F oven for 15 to 20 minutes, or until tender.

Makes 1 serving

Cooking Up a Weight-Loss Plan

LIFE IN THE FAT LANE

Even in kindergarten, Salvatore Borda was bigger than all his classmates.

"I just liked food in general," he says. "I never had a sweet tooth. It was more the meat, potatoes, and bread."

Bigness had its advantages in grade school. Kids refrain from cracking wise about a guy's weight when they know that weight may end up sitting on their sternum until they apologize.

By high school, however, the charm of being the big kid had worn off. "My football coach told me I could play fullback if I lost enough weight," he says. "But I was only able to get down to about 220 or 217."

So instead of carrying the ball, Borda ended up in the trenches, playing defensive tackle until he was sidelined with a knee injury senior year.

Life after high school revolved around food—literally. Borda entered a 2-year program at a Rhode Island culinary school and quickly fell prey to an occupational hazard: tasting too many of his own creations.

By 2000, he weighed 315 pounds and wore size-48 pants and size-triple-X sweatshirts.

The weird thing is, Borda didn't stand out at all in culinary school, where superstar chefs such as the vastly overweight Paul Prudhomme are regarded as role models. "There were a lot of people larger than me," says Borda.

Even though he looked normal in his environment, he felt bad: unquenchably thirsty, increasingly tired.

THE TURNING POINT

During a summer vacation, Borda went drinking with his father and uncles. He woke up with an unexpectedly fierce hangover and felt even worse after loading up on funnel cakes, ice cream, and cotton candy.

Suspecting he had diabetes, Borda borrowed a friend's blood-sugar testing kit—and found that his level was a horrifying 690. (A normal reading for someone who hasn't fasted is below 200.) "When I called my family doctor, he said, 'Don't even bother coming in to see me. Go straight to the hospital.'"

Tests showed that Borda had type-2, or adult-onset, diabetes—a lifestyle-related illness that's striking Americans at younger and younger ages.

"I always knew I was overweight, and I knew what I could do to fix it," he says. "I just didn't want to."

Now he had no choice.

Name: SALVATORE BORDA
Date of Birth: February 1980
Residence: Blackwood, New Jersey
Occupation: Chef
Height: 5 foot 8

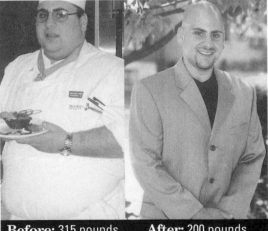

Before: 315 pounds   **After:** 200 pounds

THE PLAN OF ATTACK

Borda vowed to trim down to 225 pounds by Christmas 2000.

To help control his sky-high blood sugar, he cut out refined carbohydrates. "The only carbs I ate were vegetables and fruits," he says. He also reduced his intake of saturated fat. "I ate chicken and fish, olive oil, and nuts," he says. "For the most part, I stayed away from red meat, even though it wasn't outside my diet."

Soon after starting his diet, Borda began riding an exercise bike. At first, he could go for only 20 minutes. As his stamina improved, he increased to 55 minutes.

During the first month, he lost almost 15 pounds.

At culinary school, he learned to exercise something else: restraint. A "taste" became a taste, not a mouthful.

LIFE IN THE FIT LANE

On Christmas morning 2000, Borda weighed 226 pounds, just 1 pound above his goal. That was close enough for him to consider it a victory.

Still, he felt he could do better, so he started experimenting with different exercise routines. He began jogging, eventually working up to 5½

miles 3 or 4 days a week. He also took up bicycling. When weather permits, he goes for a 20-mile ride at least once a week. Instead of working out after he finished his 6:00-A.M.-to-2:00-P.M. shift, he started exercising at 4:00 A.M., before work.

"All my friends thought I was insane, but it put a little boost on things," he says. "Once I got pretty good at doing pushups and situps and chinups, I bought a small multistation home gym for my bedroom."

Borda's blood-sugar level had decreased, so his doctor took him off insulin shots and placed him on oral medication. As he continued to improve, his dosage was reduced twice. "I'm hoping to get off it entirely," he says.

The weight continued to burn off, and by mid-2001, Borda was under 200 pounds and wore size-32 pants. That led to one of the oddest moments of his life: He attended his sister's high school graduation and was unrecognizable to the many friends and former classmates in attendance. "Various people had found out that I had diabetes, but nobody really knew that I had lost a lot of weight," he says.

Borda quietly revealed his identity to a woman he had grad-

uated with in 1998. The woman told another female classmate that "Sal" was standing in line.

Spinning around in the line, the woman searched the crowd in vain for Borda, at one point staring straight at him. "I asked, 'Are you looking for me?' She almost fell over," says Borda.

His new self-confidence has spilled over into his social life. "That side of things has improved greatly," he says.

His new self-assurance exasperated his fellow chefs. "I'm not afraid to just stand there and tell people how good I look," he says. "People got tired of me and said, 'All right, we know. Good job. Now get back to work.'"

HIS TIPS

EDUCATE YOURSELF ABOUT HEALTHY EATING. "I met with the nutritionist in the hospital, and then afterward, one follow-up visit outside. I think my culinary knowledge and experience has helped me, too."

DON'T LET MECHANICAL FAILURES SLOW YOU DOWN. "I started with a stationary bike for about 20 minutes. Then, somewhere in February, the bike broke. I was forced to try something else. So I started walking."

Part 3
All the
Right Moves

You versus Yourself

BETTER SEX. SMALLER WAIST. IMPROVED SELF-CONFIDENCE. LONGER life. Better mood. Bigger biceps. More energy. Deeper sleep. Better concentration.

If we told you we could give you all these things, we'd sound like either the devil or that goon selling exercise machines on channel 73. (Or maybe that goon *is* the devil.)

Even if we told you we had no interest in your money (which wouldn't be entirely true, since we wanted you to buy this book) or your first-born child, you still wouldn't trust us. You'd know there must be some catch.

Indeed, there is. To get these benefits, you have to exercise— something just 15 to 20 percent of us do long enough and consistently enough to produce any health-enhancing effects.

The problem isn't that people don't understand that exercise is good for them—97 percent of us are clear on this point. And it's not that they don't try to exercise. The problem is that 50 percent of exercisers bail out within 6 months of starting an exercise program. After 21 months, the dropout rate reaches an astounding 75 percent.

Belly Busters

▶▶ "It takes a support mechanism, and mine was definitely my wife. Without her love and motivation I'm not sure I could have made it." ◀◀

—JAMES GORDON
44, LOST 60 POUNDS

Since everyone knows they're supposed to exercise yet so few people stick with it, there must be something wrong with people, something wrong with exercise, or something wrong with the way we try to get people to exercise.

Perhaps the problem is all of the above. That's the conclusion we've reached after talking with Jim Annesi, Ph.D., an exercise psychologist with the YMCA of Metropolitan Atlanta, about his groundbreaking research on the three reasons why most guys don't work out. Those reasons are:

1. Lack of self-management skills

2. Lack of social support

3. Physical discomfort

In the first two cases, there's clearly something wrong with the individuals. In the third, there's something wrong with exercise and the way we try to get people to do it. But the third, Annesi believes, is probably the most important of the three. Even if people get social support and learn to manage their time and attitudes, they won't exercise if it just freakin' hurts.

Now let's figure out why *you* aren't exercising, or why you might drop out if you are. (If you've been exercising for more than 2 years and you consider yourself at no risk of dropping out, you can skip this chapter and go straight to the exercise sections that follow. Believe us, we won't be offended.)

THE EXERCISE BALANCE SHEET

At least three studies have shown that people who create an exercise balance sheet—a cost-benefit analysis, to put it another way—are more likely to stick with exercise than those who don't. So our first goal in this chapter is to get you to put some things in writing.

Self-management skills. Think about the following skills and give yourself a letter grade—A, B, C, D, or F—in each.

▶ When the little voice in my head asks, "What's a fat slob like me doing in a gym with all these Barbie and Ken dolls?" I tell it to shut the hell up.

▶ When I tell myself I'm going to exercise three times a week no matter what, I do it. A promise is a promise, even if it's just from me to me.

▶ I'm flexible in ways that have nothing to do with stretching. If I can't exercise at the gym at 5:30, I exercise at home at 6:45. If the couch is in my way, I don't give up and sit on it—I move the damn thing.

▶ When I start to "feel the burn," I tough out the temporary discomfort.

▶ I know it'll take a while to achieve my ultimate goal of a sub-36-inch waist, so I establish smaller goals along the way and acknowledge when I've reached them.

▶ When I achieve a goal, I reward myself with a CD or a dinner at my favorite restaurant, linking material rewards to exercise adherence.

Social support. On a sheet of paper, make two columns. On the left, write down everyone who does or might support your exercise program. On the right, note all the people who don't or might not. Take into consideration your wife or girlfriend, parents, children, friends, boss, coworkers. You could even put your pet in the right-hand column if taking care of him is a constraint on your time or energy, or in the left if walking him is your best excuse to get out and burn off some chalupas.

Likes and dislikes. Make another two columns. On the left, write down what you like about exercise. On the right, record what you don't like.

INTERPRETING THE RESULTS

If most of your "Self-Management Skills" grades are C, D, and F, you let the slightest interruption throw off your workout routine, and you have problems making and acknowledging incremental gains.

The "Social Support" list is pretty easy to interpret: If the people you are closest to appear in the right-hand column, you have a discouraging lack of social support. If the major players are on the left, you don't.

If the right-hand column of your "Likes and Dislikes" list is longer than the left, you have some issues with exercise.

If a lot of your "Dislike" answers involve feeling physical discomfort during or after exercise, you're in the biggest and most difficult group of non-exercisers.

FIXING THE PROBLEMS

Each problem requires a different approach. If all three apply to you, decide which is the most serious and use the appropriate solution.

Managing yourself. Self-management is often the most prickly exercise-aversion issue. You don't hate to feel the burn, and you have plenty of support. Still, you somehow skip your workouts more often than not.

One important step is to establish clear goals and step-by-step plans to achieve them. Annesi suggests setting "outcome" goals, such as "I'm going to lose 30 pounds before my 20th reunion and make Cindy sorry that she dumped me for that skinny burnout." Other outcome goals might be to hit your drives farther or run a 10-K or bench press your own weight.

The step-by-step plans are "process" goals. They show you how you're going to reach the outcome you want. Sched-

Belly Busters

▶▶▶"All along the way, I've set goals, including to win a racquetball game, score a hockey goal, run a mile, weigh 200 pounds. I've reached every one and have progressed from 'goals' to 'dreams.' Some dreams I've reached. The others are getting closer each week."◀◀

—KEVIN SEBESTA
31, LOST 140 POUNDS

uling your workouts (we'll talk you through it in the next chapter) is an example of a process goal.

Here are the other ways you learn to manage yourself.

▶ **Stop negative thoughts.** Your brain is a magnificent trickster. It has dozens of ways to talk you out of a workout. Your best weapons are the techniques called thought stopping and cognitive restructuring. When your brain tells you not to exercise ("The boss is on the warpath and I'm too stressed to work out—we'll wait until next week"), force a rational, more positive thought into your head: "Exercise will help me relieve the stress. I'll feel worse if I don't work out this week."

▶ **Prepare for setbacks.** On the days you can't show up for your workouts, you have to employ a self-management strategy called relapse prevention. Just accept that you aren't perfect, and remind yourself that your program isn't a failure just because you missed one session. Chapter 16 will have much more detailed information about sticking with a program through a variety of inconveniences and calamities. For now, just know that everyone misses a workout from time to time, and you won't be an exception. You can and will bounce back.

▶ **Mark off the days.** After you complete a workout, mark down on your calendar what you did that day. For example, if you perform a cardiovascular exercise such as running for 20 minutes, jot down "C-20." If you complete your weight-lifting program, write "WL." If you stretch before or after, write "S." This gives you written proof of your accomplishments, which studies have shown is a strong motivation and reinforcement.

▶ **Reward yourself.** After an especially good workout, treat yourself to a whirlpool. After a week of consistent exercise, take the missus out for dinner. After a month, buy yourself a CD box set. Or simply pay yourself a dollar for every completed workout, and buy something once the money adds up. After several months of consistent regular exercise, you'll likely find you don't need to reward yourself to keep up the habit. By then your improved mood and increased energy will serve as both your reward *and* your motivation to renew that gym membership.

A long-term study of three slightly overweight men showed that self-chosen rewards helped them meet their goal of gradually increasing their walking distance by 10 percent incre-

Belly Busters

▶▶"You have to stick with it. What I did was start slow with a small number of reps. That will give you a sense of accomplishment, and then you should try to push yourself for more the next week.

"The point is to establish a routine where you will put in the time and effort. The benchmark needs to be raised constantly to avoid complacency and boredom."◀◀

—REY SIFUENTES JR.
28, LOST 91 POUNDS

ments then easing into a running program. After 2 years, the guys no longer needed tangible rewards to keep going. Exercise had become its own reward.

Enlisting social support. Some people find it tough to justify a steady, consistent exercise program. You could get hit by a bus today, they think, so what difference does it make whether you have a 35-inch waist?

This is where a strong support system comes in. A review of 113 exercise-adherence studies published in the *Journal of Sport and Exercise Psychology* shows you're more likely to make a lifetime commitment to exercise if you have some of kind social support.

The key, Annesi believes, is to feel that you're part of a group. Although you might think of yourself as the Lone Ranger, studies show that as many as 90 percent of people prefer to work out with others—either a training partner or a group such as a running club or exercise class.

We know this is a leap for a new exerciser. Why would you want to step into a health club filled with people who look like they just returned from an *MTV Spring Break* audition? Psychologists call this social physique anxiety, but you don't need eight syllables of textbook terminology to know you feel especially self-conscious when you walk into some gyms.

Here are a few strategies to help you face down the fear.

▶ Try the YMCA or another place that doesn't cater to people who already exercise regularly or have most

Belly Busters

▶▶ "I started going to my local gym, where I met the woman who changed my life: my personal trainer. A beauty named Elaine, she called me over and told me that my workouts were 'pussy.' She took me in and molded me.

"Since then, I've unlocked potential I never knew I had. I even have abs! I've put on about 25 pounds of lean muscle mass, and my body-fat percentage is about 9 percent. I even placed first in a power-lifting competition—the first trophy I've ever gotten. I show some 'before' pictures to people, and they can't believe the difference. I joke that I sometimes trip over people's dropped jaws." ◀◀

—MICHAEL SCHIDLOW
22, LOST 38 POUNDS

of the results they're going to get. Some guys may find it inspiring to be around dedicated, fit individuals (or at least pleasantly distracting to be around dedicated, fit women). But for guys who feel bad about their own appearance, spending an hour a day with chiseled, denuded barbell-heads makes corpulence seem noble by comparison.

▶ Join a private gym, where there are never more than a few people working out at a time, all with personal trainers. Tell your trainer or the gym owner that you're interested in finding one or more workout partners.

▶ Ask your doctor if he knows of any group you can join—support group, exercise program, walking club—to link up with others who share your desire to get back in shape.

▶ Support someone else. Let a coworker know that you notice he's lost a few pounds. If you know he's been training, ask how his program is going. You'll establish a common interest in weight loss and exercise, and you'll give him positive feedback that he may not be getting anywhere else. You may end up with a training partner.

▶ Hire a trainer to work with you and a buddy simultaneously. The trainer will not only provide expert instruction but also make you and your pal feel that the gym is a more normal environment for you.

One mistake a lot of guys make is hiring a trainer and relying exclusively on him or her for positive feedback. Annesi believes you can become so dependent that you can barely move a muscle without the trainer's encouragement. Trainers are good for starting or refreshing a program, but it's important to build a degree of exercise independence.

At about the same time that you start seeing results from your fitness program, you'll also start to receive compliments. They may come from your wife or friends, or from a colleague, another exerciser, or a stranger. At first, they may sound more like insults than compliments. "You don't look like Shrek anymore! What happened?"

However they phrase it, what they really mean is, "You look great." You won't be able to survive on outside approval forever—eventually, people will stop noticing incremental improvements in your physique, and you'll have to find other motivators. But when you receive those compliments, you'll feel like the biggest swinging banana in the savannah.

Dealing with discomfort. Create a diversion to take your mind off the discomfort of exercise. Psychologists call this *dissociation*. You call it *TV*. Or *music*. Or *Pilates hotties*. Practically any distraction—even something as simple as listening to street sounds or chatting with a buddy—will help reduce boredom and frustration, and disconnect your brain from the part of your body that feels the physical exertion.

No single distraction works for everyone, and studies suggest that multiple distractions may work best to improve exercise adherence. Consider what happened when researchers assigned 56 fitness-center members to one of four groups: music only, television only, music and television, and no distractions. They found that the

Belly Busters

▶▶ "The key to my success was rewards. When I dropped a certain amount of weight, I would go out and spend money on myself and buy something that I wanted to remind myself that I deserve it. It would usually be clothes, because I dropped several sizes. I went from a tight 46 waist to a loose 38-inch waist. I would also reward myself with food sometimes. Every now and then, I would allow myself a nice dessert from the dessert menu. To keep myself in check, I would then run an extra lap around the track." ◀◀

—JONATHAN HEATON
23, LOST 95 POUNDS

music-and-television group had about half the dropout rate of the other three groups. This group also registered significantly higher gains in aerobic capacity over a 14-week period.

When you're lifting weights, using multiple distractions is more difficult—not to mention more dangerous. (Nearly one-quarter of weight-lifting injuries that require emergency-room visits are smashed fingers and toes.) Still, most gyms keep the music loud in their weight rooms.

Of course, you might find exercise so unpleasant that you can't bring yourself to set foot into the gym in the first place. If that's the case, you need more than distraction. Here's kind of a radical idea: Try pain-free exercise. In chapter 12, we'll give you a very simple cardiovascular program that begins with just 10 minutes of moderate-exertion exercise three times a week, plus 5 minutes of easy-pace warmup and cooldown. The first week of the program includes a total of an hour's worth of exercise, none of it at pain-inducing levels.

The program escalates the length and intensity of workouts from there, but if you're averse to the feelings of exertion, you don't have to increase either parameter. In fact, research shows that within a couple of months, regular exercise at almost any intensity and duration will brighten your mood. Some researchers say that this happens because exercise unleashes endorphins, serotonin, and other feel-good brain chemicals. Other researchers say it's because exercise

Belly Busters

▶▶ "At 275 pounds, the thought of me working out sounded a little like playing Russian roulette: I might get lucky; I might die. I figured my body was in shock anyway with the different eating schedule. Why punish it with running or anything too strenuous at this point? So I set my exercise calendar for 230 pounds, and when I achieved this goal, I would work that body. I hit 230 in July of that year, and in keeping my promise to myself, I began to run. I hacked, spit up, and damn near died, but nonetheless I began. It took me about a week to get to a mile without croaking, but I did. I then began aerobic kickboxing and eliminated the running. I figured it had to be a much better workout because more body parts got sore. Now I'm sitting at 215 pounds for a grand total loss of 60 pounds." ◀◀

—JAMES GORDON
44, LOST 60 POUNDS

increases your sense of self-control and provides a respite from the rat race. Whatever the reason, hundreds of studies confirm that exercise improves your state of mind. So as you begin an exercise program, remember that you'll soon reap such immediate benefits as decreased stress, fatigue, and depression, and improved energy, body image, and self-esteem.

Buffness will be nice, if and when you get there, but all these other benefits come first. And once you achieve them, you'll find it easier to push yourself. You may even discover that you actually enjoy working up a good sweat and pushing your body out of its comfort zone.

He Bypassed Health Problems

LIFE IN THE FAT LANE

When Mike Stanley reflects on the past 20 years, he realizes he never recognized his weight problem. "To be honest," he says now, "I struggled with my weight my whole life." He was at his heaviest in 1997 after a 7-month recovery from a broken ankle. In each of those months, he gained almost 6 pounds, for a grand total of 40. "I had no interest in exercising or eating right," he admits.

Despite sporting a size-42 waist, Stanley's overt quality of life didn't suffer. "I dressed well, I carried myself well, I have an outgoing personality, and I didn't have any problems making friends," he says. He was on a smooth ride. Or so he thought.

THE TURNING POINT

During a routine health insurance physical in September 2000, Stanley received some startling information: He had calcium deposits in two ar-teries, 26 percent body fat, total cholesterol of 240, and a resting heart rate in the high 60s. His doctor deadpanned, "Don't be discouraged. Being 39 years old and way out of shape, you still have plenty of time to save up for a double bypass."

"I was crushed. I mean, you think you're invincible," says Stanley. With his life in the balance, he realized it was time to get serious.

THE PLAN OF ATTACK

Encouraged by his wife, Stanley dropped by a local gym. "I hadn't been in a gym in probably 10 years," he says. Draped in size-XXL gym clothes, he hoisted himself onto an elliptical trainer. Less than 7 minutes later, he thought he was going to die. "I was bright red and sucking wind hard."

Bewildered by the state-of-the-art equipment and embarrassed by his outsize physique, Stanley found it tough to adjust. "The first few times I was in there, I wasn't feeling very confident," he admits. "But the more I was there, people would say, 'Man, you're looking great. You're losing some weight. I can tell you're working hard.'" He was hooked.

Then, Stanley changed his eating habits. He switched from three huge meals a day (typical breakfast: four to six doughnuts) to six meticulously planned smaller meals. Breakfast consists of a shake made with protein powder, instant oatmeal, banana, and flaxseed oil. Then he eats three small meals during

Name: MICHAEL STANLEY
Occupation: Owner of manufacturing business
Residence: Fort Worth, Texas
Date of Birth: September 1960
Height: 5 foot 10½

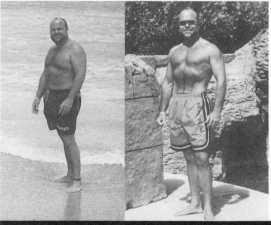

Before: 246 pounds   **After:** 170 pounds

the workday—each incorporating 5 to 6 ounces of protein, a carbohydrate, and a green vegetable. Dinner is whatever his wife prepares. "She cooks pretty healthy, but that's probably my least clean meal of the day," he says. Finally, he downs 6 ounces of pure muscle-building protein at 9:00 P.M., before he hits the sack. "On Sundays, I eat whatever I want," he adds.

Stanley's efforts paid off big-time: 14 months later, he was 76 pounds lighter.

LIFE IN THE FIT LANE
"I've changed my life completely. There are no ifs, ands, or buts about it. I just live a completely different way than I did back then," says Stanley.

Today, Stanley has a 30-inch waist to show for his efforts. "When my wife used to try to hug me, she couldn't even get her arms all the way around. Now she can touch her elbows. She says it's like she's got a brand new husband."

And his kids have a brand new dad. Before Stanley lost the weight, he'd always find an excuse not to play ball with his 7-year-old son. "Now we play football. We run. In baseball

season, I helped with his team—got out there and hit, ran the bases," says Stanley. "It's definitely enhanced our relationship." He also gets on the court with his hoops-playing daughter. "I can actually help her rather than sit in the stands and critique her," he says.

Most important, Stanley can quit saving money for that double bypass. For every pound he lost, he dropped one cholesterol point. His resting heart rate is in the low 50s, and his body fat is in the single digits: 9.7 percent. "I feel and look like a new person," he says.

HIS WORKOUT
Stanley works out 4 days a week. On Mondays, he works his back and triceps; Tuesdays, his legs; Wednesdays, his chest and biceps; Fridays, his shoulders and abs. He also does 30 minutes of cardio three to four times a week.

HIS TIPS
KEEP COMPANY. "As you start having success, people notice." You won't want to let them down.

SET A GOAL. "For my first time ever, I ran on a relay team

for the White Rock Marathon. My length was 6.2 miles, and I ran it in 53.55. A year ago, I couldn't have walked 6 miles."

LET SUCCESS MOTIVATE YOU TO STICK WITH IT. "I equate it to playing golf: If you take a golf lesson and all of a sudden you start hitting the ball better, you want to play golf all the time."

PLAN AHEAD. Stanley realized that the simple act of eating lunch took up valuable time during the day, leaving little room for workouts. "I figure I was leaving the office, driving to a restaurant, sitting down, ordering, eating, and driving back. Now I cook once a week, on Saturdays. . . . I make up a ton of meals for during the day while I'm at work. Now, I don't have any problems stealing that hour to go work out."

CONTROL YOUR TIME. "I won't schedule any lunch appointments anymore to go out and eat crappy food with a salesman."

BE CREATIVE. "In the middle of this, I went on vacation with my family. When the hotel gym wasn't open, I found myself running stairs. I got out in the water, swam with the kids, threw the Frisbee, jogged up and down the beach. I got back from the vacation, and I'd lost 8 pounds."

The Rules
for Success

OVER THE YEARS, MEN'S HEALTH HAS INTERVIEWED LITERALLY
thousands of exercise and weight-control experts. Here's a
compendium of the best advice they've given us. And if you
don't want to just take our word that these are the tips that
work, check out the "Belly-Off Success Story" profiles
throughout the book. Within those accounts of guys who've
conquered their bellies, you'll see real-life applications of these
basic workout rules.

RULE 1: DO SOMETHING

Everyone is better off incorporating some sort of exercise into their
lives on a near-daily basis. Something is always better than nothing.
Our bodies are designed for movement, so when we don't move,
our bodies fall apart.

RULE 2: DO SOMETHING YOU LIKE

If you really enjoy one type of exercise, take it on faith that it's
better for you than the alternatives. If you like it and get the benefits you want, it *is* better for you.

RULE 3: MATCH YOUR EXERCISE TO YOUR GOALS

From time to time, certain types of exercise get massively oversold to the public. Though we're all for clever marketing, some odd ideas work their way into the fitness mainstream. A perfect example is a recent TV newsmagazine story about teens getting plastic surgery. The report featured a girl who wanted liposuction. She told the reporter she had done everything she could to lose the fat around her middle. The next image was her exercising to a Tae Bo video.

Understand, Tae Bo is a perfectly fine workout system. You burn some calories, develop some flexibility, and learn how to kick and throw a punch. Tae Bo and Pilates and power yoga—and any other exercise system that lends itself to video series and overflowing workout studios—work for rules 1 and 2, which are the most important. You're doing something, and you're doing something you enjoy. But is this the type of exercise you would choose if you were doing *everything* you could to lose weight?

Absolutely not. If you want to burn a significant number of calories, you'd choose straight aerobic exercise, such as running or cycling or rowing. If you want to build muscle and thus speed up your metabolism, you'd choose strength training.

For what it's worth, the girl in the TV report got her surgery. She transformed herself from a fat girl with a bulging midsection to a fat girl with a flat

Belly Busters

▶▶"I look forward to going to the gym every night. Before, I would find myself in a bar after work for 2 hours."◀◀

—FRANK SERAFINI
30, LOST 80 POUNDS

middle. And it made her happy, which is worth something. But if only she had found an exercise program better matched to her goals, she would have been able to look better everywhere.

RULE 4: HARDER IS BETTER THAN EASIER

About 10 years ago, walking began being touted as a weight-loss strategy. New studies showed the life-extending benefits of moderate exercise, and experts were promoting it like crazy. Hey, why bother getting all tired and sweaty? Just walk and you'll lose weight, live longer, think better, and on and on.

And walking can indeed be a great strategy for following rules 1 and 2: If all you'll do is walk and you won't do anything if you don't walk, go out and take a nice long stroll. Don't let us talk you out of it.

But if you think it's as good as a run for weight loss, don't kid yourself. Sure, walking burns a few calories, but not as many as you could expend in half the time with intense exercise.

See, submaximal exercise—walking, slow cycling, anything that doesn't take you out of your comfort zone—turns

Belly Busters

▶▶ "I have been doing a workout I found on the Internet: Day 1—all the pushups I can do. Day 2—all the situps I can do. Day 3—2 sets of pullups, 3 sets of situps, and 3 sets of pushups. Day 4—all the pullups I can do. Day 5—rest. Day 6—start all over with Day 1." ◀◀

—JON ZIEGLER
38, LOST 25 POUNDS

up your metabolism while you're doing it. But intense exercise, such as running or weight lifting, keeps your metabolism running at a higher speed after you're finished. In the case of weight lifting, that metabolic increase could last 48 hours. There's less of an afterburn with running and other types of aerobic exercise, but you tend to burn more calories during those activities than you do while lifting weights, so in the end it's probably safe to say that any type of intense exercise is better for weight loss and overall health than any type of easy exercise.

In fact, Canadian researchers have found that high-intensity interval training is nine times better for fat loss than long, slow endurance exercise. (Don't worry, we'll tell you how to do interval training in chapter 11.)

Furthermore, a 2001 study in *Obesity Research* found that overweight men get even *less* out of submaximal exercise after losing weight. Everyone should start into exercise slowly and gradually build up strength and endurance. But once you're in shape,

you have to make exercise more challenging, or you'll quickly learn the most dreaded phrase in the fitness world: *diminishing returns*.

RULE 5: WHENEVER POSSIBLE, EXERCISE SHOULD BE USEFUL

One of the buzzwords among trainers today is *functional*. If an exercise improves your body in a way that helps you perform your daily activities with less pain and more efficiency, it's considered functional. If it doesn't, it isn't.

When you take a hard look at many popular exercises, you realize they don't pass the functionality test. For example, many guys who lift weights obsess over their maximum bench press—how much weight they can push off their chest one time while lying on a bench. But if you try to attach a real-life application to a maximum bench press, you'll probably fail.

Likewise, endurance running is one of the most revered fitness activities. If you go to a sports-medicine conference, you'll find the streets thick morning, noon, and night with jogging doctors and researchers. Aerobic exercise has more benefits than we can list here, but it's hard to argue that training your body to run, ride, or swim long distances is particularly useful. When in real life do you need to run farther than the distance from your front door to the bus station?

What's useful depends on the user, of course, but it doesn't hurt to ask the following questions if you're in doubt about an exercise.

▶ **"Does it improve strength, speed, power, or coordination in a way that applies to my life?"** Take the deadlift, for example, an exercise in which you lift a heavy weight off the floor. To do it well and without injury, you have to learn to keep your back in a safe, stable position and lift the weight with your powerful lower-body muscles. That's one of the most useful exercises imaginable, since the basic skill of lifting an inert object (garbage can, sleeping child, passed-out drinking buddy) constantly comes in handy.

▶ **"Does it increase my flexibility in a useful way, or hinder it?"** We don't mean to pick on yoga here, since a lot of people enjoy it and find that it helps take the edge off the stress of daily life. But while some flexibility is good, lotus-position flexibility doesn't prepare you for any real-world challenges.

On the other hand, some types of exercise hinder flexibility. Running, for example, is notorious for creating tight hamstring, calf, and lower-back muscles. Weight lifting with poor form or unbalanced exercise selection can have the same effect. Many guys lift weights through a shortened range of motion because they're able to lift more that way. But the affected muscles can grow tighter and, in effect, shorten themselves. Similarly, many guys like to develop their chest muscles but don't spend equal time and energy on their middle-back muscles. The resulting imbalance of strength can compromise posture.

▶ **"If hell lands on my doorstep, is there any part of my exercise program I'll be glad I did?"** Could you carry your wife or kids out of a burning house? Sprint away from an attacker? Overpower and disarm him? Not many of us are confronted with these situations (thankfully), but if you stop to think about it, the same exercises that prepare us for life-or-death emergencies also help us play sports better, do heavy yard work, and open pickle jars for our wives.

Belly Busters

▶▶ "The first and foremost thing that helped me was just getting up every morning and telling myself that I was a changed man—training my mind to believe it. Next came enormous self-discipline. I had to tell myself every day that I needed to work out and what I had to gain if I stayed true to my plan.

"The workouts started with basic pushups and situps three times a week, once per day. I moved to 5 days a week and then included dips between chairs, pullups, calf raises, and more ab routines. I started to play basketball and Ultimate Frisbee three or four times a week as well.

"Now, 6 months later, I lift weights 4 evenings a week, run 3 days a week for 15 to 60 minutes, and start the mornings with my pushups and ab workouts."◀◀

—STERLING RASKIE
25, LOST 55 POUNDS

RULE 6: YOU DON'T HAVE TO DO EVERYTHING

Twenty to 60 minutes of aerobic exercise a day, 3 to 5 days a week. A half-hour of strength training, 2 or 3 days a week. Five to 10 minutes of stretching, 2 or 3 days a week.

A serious training program for advanced athletes? No, these are exercise *minimums* recommended by the American College of Sports Medicine.

Ignore, for a moment, the improbability that anyone would ever do all this. The real issue is: Why would anyone want to?

If you like to run, run. Weight lifting can make you a better runner, but I doubt you'd need 1 to 1½ hours of lifting a week to benefit. Three 15-minute sessions a week should do it.

If you like to lift, lift. Aerobic exercise probably won't do anything to make you a better lifter, although it can certainly help you burn off some extra fat. Worse, if you do a lot of aerobic exercise, you negate some of the benefits of strength training. There's a well-known, though not well-understood, interference effect that occurs when someone tries to develop serious strength and aerobic endurance at the same time: You don't put on muscle or build strength as fast as you would without the aerobics. (Curiously, the lifting doesn't limit aerobic gains.)

So a guy who's doing serious strength exercise—at least 3 hours of intense lifting per week—needs zero aerobic exercise, although two or three short sessions per week probably won't hurt and should help burn off fat. But if you like lifting and hate aerobics, you don't ever need to lace up those running shoes.

As for the American College of Sports Medicine's stretching recommendations, they may be superfluous for weight lifters. Lifting through a full range of motion should maintain or even slightly increase your flexibility, so stretching probably isn't necessary.

On the other hand, most runners incorporate stretching into their routines, usually after a run. For them, it's probably necessary. As explained above, endurance exercise hampers flexibility, making muscles shorter and tighter through repetitive, short-range movements. So a guy who does one type of aerobic exercise 3 to 5 hours a week will almost certainly do himself a massive favor by stretching seriously for 5 to 10 minutes most days.

Belly Busters

▶▶▶ "My exercise routine first started out as walking, then progressed to biking, and after 70 pounds of weight loss, I hit the gym." ◀◀◀

—JOEY CALLAWAY
26, LOST 185 POUNDS

RULE 7: FROM TIME TO TIME, IGNORE RULES 2 THROUGH 6

A guy who's been exercising a while gets into certain grooves, or ruts. (Someone more clever than we are once said the difference between the two is the depth.) He may be doing what he enjoys most. He may be doing exactly what he needs to build muscle or burn fat, whichever is his major goal. He may be doing exercise that's both intense and useful. And he may have successfully ignored the fitness establishment's admonition to do everything, focusing instead on what he needs and enjoys.

And yet, that guy may find he's stopped improving in the areas he cares about. His weight isn't decreasing or his waist isn't shrinking or his shoulders aren't widening.

Or maybe he just doesn't enjoy his workouts the way he used to.

Someday, you will be that guy. Becoming that guy is a good thing. It means you've exercised so long and so hard and so consistently that you've derived all the physical or psychological benefits you're going to get from your current exercise model.

You need to try something new. That could mean shifting from a type of workout you enjoy to something you think you'll dislike. It could mean switching to exercises that aren't perfectly matched to your goals or that aren't all that useful. It might mean adding aerobics to a weight-lifting program, or adding weights to an aerobic program.

And the changes may not help.

But you can't know what they'll accomplish until you try them.

MIX 'EM, MATCH 'EM, TRADE 'EM WITH YOUR FRIENDS

Now that you understand the rules, it's time to shift from theory to prac-

Belly Busters

▶▶ "I have had trouble isolating my biceps. I found one exercise that gives me the deep biceps burn I was looking for: I stand with my back and elbows against the wall and perform the biceps curl that way." ◀◀

—DAVID RICHARDSON
42, LOST 60 POUNDS

tice and decide how to shape your workout to shape up your body. We recommend a three-step process.

1. Choose your main activity. Though there are hundreds of possibilities, your specific goal of losing your gut narrows them down considerably. For the sake of simplicity, pick one of two activities: strength training and aerobic exercise.

Made your choice? Good. Let's move on.

2. Select a time and place. Home or gym? Street or track? Local park or local college? Mornings or evenings? Before breakfast or after? Right after work, or a couple hours after dinner?

Don't be vague here. If you aren't decisive about where and when you're going to exercise, the chance you'll actually work out is about zero.

3. Schedule your workouts. Pull out your calendar and write in every workout you plan to do for the duration of your program—all 8 or 10 or 12 weeks. Once you have a program (there are sample strength and aerobic programs in the next two chapters), mark the days when an important variable will change: the first workout in which you'll attempt speed drills, if you're a runner; or the weight-lifting session in which you'll add an extra set to each exercise.

If you've never followed a specific program before, this may seem excessively regimented. Once you try it, you'll probably find that changes are stimulating and motivating. If you don't like a particular phase of a program, you can count down the workouts until it ends. (Doing something you dislike violates Rule 2 but makes sense when you've been working out long enough for Rule 7 to kick in.) If there's a type of workout that you enjoy more than others, you look forward to the week when you can start doing it.

4. Figure out how you're going to make progress. When you get to the sample programs in the next two chapters, you'll see that each requires more total work each week, as well as harder work. So progress is built into the programs. No matter which program you choose—one of those, or one someone else designed—progress is a crucial element. Make sure you know exactly how the program works to build the strength and stamina you need to reach your goals.

5. Determine how you'll judge progress. If your goal is to lose weight, you simply weigh yourself, right? And if your goal is to shrink your gut, you measure your gut. Does it get any simpler than that?

No, it doesn't get simpler, but those two tests may not give you a true measure of your progress. Weight loss is a complex process; in our experience, progress is rarely linear. Sometimes weight comes off quickly and then hits a plateau. Sometimes your waist shrinks quickly but your weight doesn't change a lot. Sometimes you make substantial progress in strength or aerobic fitness without losing much weight or belly fat.

And then there's the win-the-battle, lose-the-war scenario: Maybe you lose weight quickly, but your strength doesn't improve, indicating you may be losing a lot of muscle. We've already noted that rapid muscle loss can lead to a slowed metabolism and a weight regain that's mostly fat—making you worse off than if you'd never tried to lose weight.

It's critical, in other words, to have additional ways to measure progress. Here are some possibilities.

Photo. Take a picture once a month in the same pose, wearing the same pair of shorts, standing sideways in front of the same bare wall, using the same lighting. Don't push out anything for the first picture or suck in

Belly Busters

▶▶▶"I hit the gym every morning before work. At first, it was extremely hard getting myself out of bed that early and [getting] motivated to exercise. Then I found a buddy to make me get up and lift with him every morning. This was the best thing a friend could do for me."◀◀◀

—JONATHAN COLEMAN
25, LOST 39 POUNDS

anything for subsequent pictures. You want an accurate comparison.

Body fat. Measure your waist (at the narrowest point, just under your belly button) and your hips (at the widest point, around your rear end). Divide your waist by your hips to get your waist-hip ratio. Do this every month. You want this number to shrink as you progress.

A smaller waist in proportion to your hips means you're losing belly fat without losing muscle. Bigger hips in relation to your waist most likely means you're gaining muscle. A smaller waist with smaller hips means you're probably losing muscle along with fat. And a bigger waist with smaller hips means either you're doing everything wrong or you have a medical condition that you need to address.

Strength. You don't need to test your maximum bench press or anything like that to see if you're getting stronger. Simply keep track of how much weight you're using for basic exercises. If you start out using 50 pounds on the lat-pulldown machine and after a month you're using 70 for the same number of repetitions, you have some proof. Another good measure is the number of pullups you can do. If you go from zero to two the first month, from two to five the second month, and from five to eight the third month, that's phenomenal progress.

Another fun measure, if you like math, is to total all the weight you lift in each workout. That is, sets multiplied by repetitions, multiplied by amount of

Belly Busters

▶▶"I started a log to record my weight and had a friend take a picture of me. I had my own 'before' picture, and now it was up to me to get to the 'after' picture."◀◀

—JONATHAN COLEMAN
25, LOST 39 POUNDS

weight lifted. If you lifted an average of 8,000 pounds each workout one week, 8,400 in the next week's workouts, and 9,000 the next, you know you're increasing your total work significantly and systematically. It's hard to brag about these numbers around the water cooler, since no one else will understand their importance. But it's cool to see such measurable improvement.

Endurance. Cardio athletes can measure their progress two ways: how far they go and how fast they go. Track your miles or your speeds in a training log or on your calendar, and it's easy to see how much progress you're making.

Some numbers to track:

▶ Total time spent exercising each week

▶ Total miles per week

▶ Average distance per run

▶ Length (in time or miles) of longest run each week

▶ Your speed at any given distance

▶ Number of speed intervals completed

Belly Busters

▶▶ "The journal I keep reminds me of the progress I have made and serves as motivation by inspiring me to continue my progress and set new goals."◀◀

—RAFFAEL BORELLI
34, LOST 40 POUNDS

6. Make a commitment. The first 6 months to a year of an exercise program are the toughest part. Statistically, about half of all exercisers drop out of a program within this window. So you need a way to get through this crucial period without quitting.

Our advice: Take it 4 weeks at a time.

That is, on the first day of the month, write down every workout you plan to perform that month. As suggested earlier, also write down specific goals of your workouts for the month. Let's say you've chosen running as your primary fitness activity. And let's say Sunday is your "long" day—your farthest run of the week. On each Sunday of your calendar, write down a specific target distance.

The first day of the next month, do the same thing: Commit to 4 weeks' worth of workouts, with specific goals noted on specific days.

Don't write down a workout on a day you know you won't do it. If you know you'll be working late one evening or attending a happy hour another afternoon, you won't be able to squeeze in after-work exercise sessions on those days. So don't bother writing them down. Find other days for them.

You'll have to adjust your workout schedule as the month progresses, simply because circumstances always change. When that happens, erase the affected workout and find another place for it on your calendar.

What you can't allow yourself to do, except in a true emergency, is skip a workout altogether. If you can't make it one day, you have to find a way to squeeze it in another time.

The Picture of Success

LIFE IN THE FAT LANE

Not so long ago, the click of a camera made Mark Meador shudder. "I used to hate having pictures taken," he says. Every time he found himself in the crosshairs of a photographer's lens, he'd block the shot with his outstretched hand. "It was because of my weight."

A high school track star, Meador's weight problem didn't begin until he graduated and quit running. He didn't quit eating the foods he loved: daily 12-packs of Little Debbie snack cakes and six-packs of soda, platefuls of greasy fried foods, super-size breakfasts. Without the discipline of regular exercise, all those calories slowly coalesced into a super-size belly. He tipped the scales at 207 pounds just 8 years after marching to "Pomp and Circumstance" in his high school gym.

Attempting to shed the weight, Meador crunched his abs thousands of times, logged hundreds of running miles, ate gallons of ramen-noodle soup. A martial arts fanatic, he even signed up for karate classes. At one point, he got his weight as low as 175. "I thought I was pretty trim then, so I just stopped doing it," he says.

Each time he stopped exercising, the pounds crept back.

THE TURNING POINT

One day in May 2001, Meador's 3-year-old daughter pointed to his gut and asked, "Daddy, are you having a baby?"

"I laughed at the time, but inside I was crushed," he says.

To make things worse, a visiting buddy saw some recent vacation photos of him. "Man," the friend wisecracked, "you look like Big Pun."

It was his wake-up call: In the space of a day, he'd been likened to a pregnant woman and an obese rapper who died at 28 of a heart attack. "That day, I knew I had to do something about my weight," he says.

(continued)

Name: MARK MEADOR
Occupation: Corporate recruiter for Nationwide Insurance
Residence: Westerville, Ohio
Date of Birth: November 1965
Height: 5 foot 8

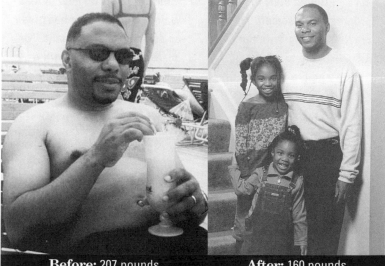

Before: 207 pounds   **After:** 160 pounds

THE PLAN OF ATTACK

"I would always see infomercials about Tae Bo, so I purchased the package," says Meador. Tae Bo, a workout developed by trainer Billy Blanks, borrows from martial arts by combining aerobics with self-defense techniques including kicking and punching. For Meador, it was the perfect mix. "I'm not a sales rep for Tae Bo, but it's kind of addicting," he says.

And Meador finally figured out the best way to keep himself on a fitness program: He exercised first thing in the morning. "When I joined the karate class, it met three times a week, during the evenings," he says. "I would start to make progress, and something would come up with the kids. I'd have to miss practices—and the weight started coming back on." Now, upon waking up every morning, Meador pops in his Tae Bo tape, and by 6:30 A.M., he's worked up his daily sweat.

Meador also ditched the fried foods, favoring baked or grilled meats, soups, and lots of fruits, vegetables, whole grains, nuts, and yogurt. As for his snack-cake habit, he reduced his support of the Little Debbie corporation: He's down to 1 cake a day, instead of 12. In the first week that Meador started his program, he lost 8 pounds; after 4 months, 39 pounds.

LIFE IN THE FIT LANE

Meador used to suffer from chronic headaches, a fact he attributes to his poor diet and high sugar intake. "When I changed my diet and stopped drinking all the pop, I stopped getting headaches," he says.

No one is more impressed by his success than his coworkers, many of whom have asked him for instructions on how to lose weight. His daughter has given up asking if he's pregnant. "Oh, no. Now she's joking with my wife, who actually is pregnant," he says.

And he no longer has reason to be camera shy. "On vacations, I can easily take my shirt off," says Meador.

HIS WORKOUT

For weight loss, Meador did an hour of Tae Bo six mornings a week. Today, he does just a half-hour, for maintenance. He also does 500 situps a day. Three times a week, he does strength training consisting of 3 60-second sets of each of the following exercises: dumbbell squat, dumbbell bench press, one-arm dumbbell row, standing lateral raise with dumbbells, and barbell triceps extension.

HIS TIPS

ESTABLISH A ROUTINE. "I wake up at 5:30 every morning, so it's easy not to fall out of the morning workout habit."

LET YOURSELF CHEAT. "I still eat my Little Debbie chocolate gels every day—but only one now, never the whole box. And especially on the weekends, I allow myself a cheat day: maybe a pancake breakfast or a pizza night."

GO FOR HALF-FARE. "At restaurants, you always feel bad if you don't eat everything, because you spent the money. So you force yourself to eat it all. Lately when my wife and I go out to eat, instead of ordering two entrées, we order one and split it in half."

Lift Weights to Lose Weight

REGARDLESS OF THEIR WEIGHT, AFTER ABOUT AGE 30 MEN TEND TO lose muscle mass rapidly. This has bigger implications than just making us look ridiculous in swimsuits. The more muscle we lose, the slower our metabolisms become. The slower our metabolisms, the easier it is to accumulate body fat. The more fat we put on, the more vulnerable we are to a long string of health problems, from heart disease to diabetes and everything else we hashed out in chapter 3. As we get weaker and fatter, our self-esteem plummets, making a comeback even more difficult.

Thankfully, there is a way to fight back. A solid, consistent weight-lifting program increases strength and muscle mass, which increases metabolism, which leads to less body fat. Strength training also improves insulin action, as shown in a 2001 study in the *Journal of the American Geriatrics Society*. Other studies have shown that strength training improves glucose uptake into muscles. (To be fair, aerobic exercise also has this effect on glucose.) Improvements in insulin action and glucose uptake can reduce your risk of diabetes.

Some studies have shown that strength training can improve your levels of "good" (HDL) cholesterol. This effect seems to depend on the type of program used. If you do high repetitions with light weights, you could see increased HDL levels. If you use heavier weights for fewer repetitions, you probably won't see any change.

A 1992 study found that weight training speeded up the transit of food through your digestive system by as much as 56 percent, and that could reduce your risk of colon cancer. Other research has shown strength training to improve blood pressure—not enormously but enough to modify health risks.

All of these benefits come into play when you're trying to lose weight. For example, improved insulin function and glucose metabolism may mean less fatigue. A reduction in blood pressure means you can work harder with less risk of overloading your cardiovascular system. And research shows that weight training particularly works to help you lose weight where you most want to. For example, in a 1996 study, strength training coupled with diet changes produced a 40 percent reduction in belly fat in obese middle-age men.

BIG NEWS FOR BIG GUYS

In this chapter, we're going to make some assumptions, examine some pre-liminary research, and then take a few flying leaps into the scientific unknown.

We're going to assume you're a naturally big guy—big arms, big legs, big shoulders, and unfortunately, a big belly. And we're going to assume that underneath your fat, you have some big muscles, or potentially big muscles.

We base these assumptions on a study presented in 2001 at the annual meeting of the North American Association for the Study of Obesity. In that study, 12 pairs of identical twins were deliberately overfed for 100 days. The pairs who had the highest proportion of type-II muscle fibers were the ones who gained the most fat. Conversely, the twins with higher proportions of type-I muscle fibers gained the least.

Stay with us as we explain the importance of this: Type-II muscle fibers are called fast-twitch, meaning they're responsible for quick bursts of energy. They're the key fibers for lifting heavy weights. They're also the ones with the most potential for growth. In other words, these are the fibers that turn a guy into a big guy.

Type-I muscle fibers are called slow-twitch; they allow you to work continuously for long periods of time, as in aerobic exercise.

The idea that everyone's muscles are basically the same is one of the key assumptions made by one-size-fits-all exercise and diet programs. As the twins study shows, your predominant muscle-fiber type makes a big difference in how you should eat. We would argue that it also shows which type of exercise will be most productive for you.

In any given weight-lifting study, results vary wildly. Some people gain strength and muscle mass as if they were on steroids; others don't show much improvement. So it was logical for researchers to do a study in which they divided their subjects into groups according to overall build—thinner or thicker. They found that the more slender guys didn't get much benefit from weight lifting. The guys who were bigger to begin with got the results you'd expect—in this case, each gained about 3½ pounds of muscle in 12 weeks of training.

Let's add up the implications of these two studies.

1. Guys who have a higher proportion of slow-twitch fibers are less likely to gain fat from overeating.

2. Guys with more slow-twitch fibers have a natural advantage in endurance activities and sports—they're better at those than are the Clydesdales lumbering along with all that heavy muscle and fat.

3. Guys with more slender builds—who probably have a higher proportion of slow-twitch fibers and a lower proportion of fast-twitch fibers—don't get particularly good results from strength training.

In sum: Guys who are naturally slender, and who are naturally suited for aerobic exercise, don't put on weight—fat or muscle—easily.

Now here's the part about you.

1. Guys who have a higher proportion of fast-twitch fibers are more likely to gain fat from overeating.

2. Guys who have more fast-twitch fibers have a natural disadvantage in aerobic activities. Their bodies aren't designed for it and won't respond as well to it.

3. Guys with bigger builds have a natural advantage in strength training—they get results fast.

In sum: Guys who are naturally big—who put on weight easily—get the best exercise results from strength training, rather than aerobic exercise.

We made some leaps of science and logic to put together this argument, but you have to admit it makes sense based on what all of us have seen with our own eyes. How come skinny runner guys can eat whatever they want? Well, possibly because they have no natural propensity to gain fat in the first place. How come you see so many weight lifters with big guts? Possibly because the kind of guy who responds well to strength training also has a tendency to put on fat easily.

Now that we've made the argument and kinda-sorta defended it, let's forget about it for the rest of this chapter. If you enjoy aerobic exercise and don't care for strength training, that's fine. We won't be offended if you don't jump into the weight-training program that follows. We just want big guys to realize that endurance exercise may not be the best choice for them, all else being equal.

(By the way, neither strength training nor aerobics will help you lose much weight if you don't cut the calories in your diet, which we showed you how to do in chapter 8.)

THE 8-WEEK BELLY-OFF WEIGHT-TRAINING PROGRAM

The goal of this training program designed by Canadian certified strength-and-conditioning coach Craig Ballantyne, C.S.C.S., is to increase energy expenditure while building muscle. Successful weight loss via weight training is a combination of those two elements. You need to burn calories to lose weight now, and you need to build muscle to increase your metabolism and prevent weight gain in the future.

The program: Every week, do three workouts with at least a day in between. (A Monday-Wednesday-Friday schedule works as well as anything.) The sample program includes three total-body workouts, each of which you do once a week.

If you've never lifted, or if you've been away from it for awhile, you have to rely on trial and error to determine the amount of weight you'll lift in each exercise. Try to increase the amount of weight you use by about 10 percent each week.

Circuits versus straight sets: The first two workouts are circuit-type programs. That means you do 1 set of each exercise in the routines before doing a second set of any exercise. The third workout consists of straight sets, in which you do 3 sets of an exercise before moving on to the next exercise.

Circuits eliminate wasted time between sets. When you move from exercise to exercise, you get more work done in less time. Plus, each muscle group gets several minutes to recover before it gets worked again. That allows you to work it more intensely each time through the circuit.

Belly Busters

▶▶ "Two days before my 30th birthday, I took a good look in the mirror and realized it wasn't the shirt or the jeans that made me look fat—it was the gut I was stuffing in them. I joined Gold's Gym that afternoon and started working out.

"In 5 months, I have gone from a 44½-inch waist to a 34. I also have gone from 240 pounds on a 5-foot-11 frame to 190 pounds." ◀◀

—RON ROSSI
31, LOST 55 POUNDS

Straight sets, on the other hand, force you to exhaust each muscle group thoroughly before you move on to the next one. That exhaustion provokes the muscles to make adaptations so they're better able to handle the workload the next time you train them.

Warmups: Whether you're doing circuits or straight sets, always start with a warmup set of each exercise. This is crucial to the success of the program. The warmup doesn't just literally warm up your muscles and joints; it also prepares your nervous system for the coming work.

When you do circuits, start with a warmup circuit using one-half to two-thirds of the weight you'll use in your work circuits: Choose a weight you can lift about 20 times, but do only 10 to 12 repetitions.

Use the same formula when warming up for straight sets: 1 to 3 sets of 6 to 12 repetitions with a weight you could lift about 20 times. After doing your warmup sets of a particular exercise, rest for a minute before beginning your first work set of that exercise.

What to expect: Doing three different workouts, each consisting of different exercises, each week ensures that your body will take a while to get used to the program. Your muscles will have to work hard to adapt to the exercises. At first, the adaptations will be mostly neurological: Your nerves

Belly Busters

▶▶ "By the time I graduated college, in May 2000, I'd really let myself go. I had become much less active, and the extra pounds just crept on month after month.

"My first real job was a desk job. Fast-food lunches and dinners added to my weight and overall fatigue. I was in my early 20s and felt like I was in my 40s.

"In December of that year, I decided that enough was enough. I spent the last 2 weeks in December making a few simple goals for the new year: I wanted to lose 30 pounds by my 24th birthday, which was 12 weeks away.

"The 12 weeks cruised by, and the pounds cruised away, too. I lost 36 pounds. I felt a great sense of accomplishment and impressed a few friends, too.

"I now have a pattern started that I am not willing to change for the world. I've gained muscle mass, energy, and confidence! I feel 20 times better." ◀◀

—JONATHAN COLEMAN
25, LOST 39 POUNDS

and muscles will get better at working together to move the weights more efficiently. You'll get stronger, but your muscles probably won't get bigger. While muscle growth occurs after only one training session, it won't be visible for weeks. Expect visible results after about 4 weeks of steady training, depending on your body-fat levels.

Fat loss, on the other hand, will be apparent much sooner. As soon as you start expending more calories than you take in, you'll start burning your body's stored fat for energy. Your metabolism will kick into a higher gear, burning more calories in between workouts as well as during them. With the dietary changes in chapter 8, plus this exercise program, you could lose a pound or two of fat each week for 8 weeks.

This will create a stunning change in your appearance, even if the difference doesn't seem that impressive when you stand on a scale. And you should feel like a new man on the inside, too.

WORKOUT 1

Start with a warmup circuit, as described earlier. Then do 10 repetitions of each exercise in a circuit—that is, do 1 set of every exercise on this list. (That's called a circuit.) Then go through and do them again—another circuit—if you want. If you're a total beginner, or you haven't exercised in months, aim for one circuit the first week or two, and build up to three circuits by the sixth or seventh week.

Each week, try to increase the amount of weight you use by about 10 percent. Make a fresh photocopy of this training log and take it to the gym with you. Record the amount of weight you use for each move and the number of repetitions you complete.

Exercise	Circuit 1		Circuit 2		Circuit 3	
	Wt	Reps	Wt	Reps	Wt	Reps
Barbell squat						
Barbell or dumbbell bench press						
45-degree traveling lunge with dumbbells						
Wide-grip seated row						
Farmer's walk on toes with dumbbells						
Swiss-ball crunch						

WORKOUT 2

Do a warmup circuit followed by 15 repetitions of each exercise in a circuit. After a few weeks, you can do a second circuit, if you choose, but this workout will be most productive if you work as hard as you can for one circuit.

Each week, try to increase the amount of weight you use by about 10 percent. Make a fresh photocopy of this training log and take it to the gym with you. Record the amount of weight you use for each move and the number of repetitions you complete.

Exercise	Circuit 1		Circuit 2 (optional)	
	Wt	Reps	Wt	Reps
Leg press				
Wide-grip barbell bench press				
Good morning				
Towel pulldown				
45-degree lying dumbbell row				
Towel crunch				

WORKOUT 3

Do 3 consecutive sets of 10 repetitions of each exercise, following a warmup set, before moving on to the next exercise. (In other words, this isn't a circuit routine.)

Each week, try to increase the amount of weight you use by about 10 percent. Make a fresh photocopy of this training log and take it to the gym with you. Record the amount of weight you use for each move and the number of repetitions you complete.

Exercise	Set 1		Set 2		Set 3	
	Wt	Reps	Wt	Reps	Wt	Reps
Dumbbell split squat						
Wide-grip stiff-legged deadlift						
Barbell or dumbbell bench press						
One-arm lat pulldown						
Twisting dumbbell shoulder press						
Bridge						

WORKOUT 1

Barbell Squat

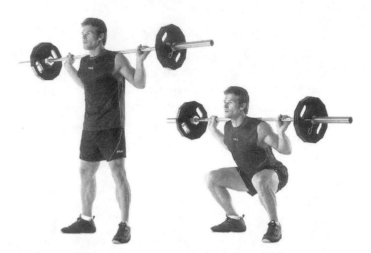

▶ Stand holding a barbell evenly across your shoulders and upper back muscles (not on your neck). Set your feet shoulder-width apart, and bend your knees slightly. Keep your lower back in its naturally arched position.

▶ Push your hips backward, and bend your knees until your upper thighs are slightly below parallel to the floor.

▶ Stand back up to the starting position.

▶ *If you're a beginner:* Try it without a barbell. Hold your arms straight out in front of you. If that's comfortable, place your hands on your hips for the next set. Then hold your hands behind your head as if you were doing a situp. When that's comfy, try it with a very light barbell.

Barbell or Dumbbell Bench Press

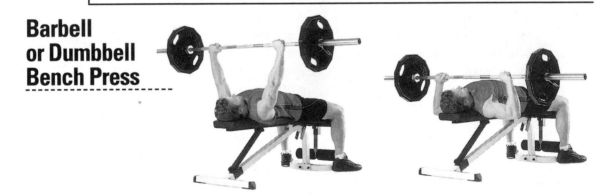

▶ Lie on a bench, and grab a barbell overhanded, your hands as wide as if you were doing a pushup—you want the action at your shoulders to feel as natural as possible. Hold the bar over your chest with your arms straight. Plant your feet flat on the floor.

▶ Or, grab a pair of dumbbells and hold them with straight arms over your chest.

▶ Slowly lower the bar to your chest or the dumbbells to the sides of your chest. Avoid arching your back or bouncing the bar off your chest.

▶ Push back up to the starting position.

▶ *If you're a beginner:* Do the exercise as described.

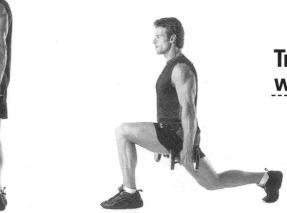

45-Degree Traveling Lunge with Dumbbells

▶ Hold a pair of dumbbells at your sides with an overhand grip, and stand someplace where you can take about 10 steps forward without annoying anybody.

▶ With your left leg, take a large step out at a 45-degree angle, lowering yourself until your left thigh is parallel to the floor and your right knee is nearly touching the floor. Your torso should stay upright.

▶ Stand up, bringing your right foot up next to your left.

▶ With your right leg, lunge forward at a 45-degree angle, then stand as you bring your left foot forward to meet your right.

▶ Lunge five times with each leg, then turn around and repeat.

▶ *If you're a beginner:* Try this without weights until you master the movement.

Wide-Grip Seated Row

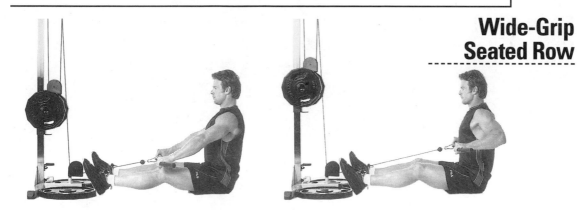

▶ Attach a straight bar to a low cable, brace your feet against the footrest, and bend your knees slightly. Grab the bar with an overhand grip, and sit upright with your lower back in its natural alignment. Pull your shoulders back to their natural position, and start the exercise with your arms nearly straight.

▶ Pull the bar to your lower abdomen.

▶ Slowly return the bar to the starting position.

▶ *If you're a beginner:* Use a very light weight and do the exercise as described.

Farmer's Walk on Toes with Dumbbells

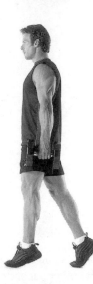

▶ Grab a pair of dumbbells with an overhand grip, hold them at your sides, and stand wherever you stood for the 45-degree traveling lunge with dumbbells.

▶ Rise up on your toes, and walk forward 10 steps with each leg. Stay on your toes the entire time.

▶ Turn and walk back 10 steps with each leg.

▶ *If you're a beginner:* Try the exercise without weights at first. If it's easy, use weights on the next set.

Swiss-Ball Crunch

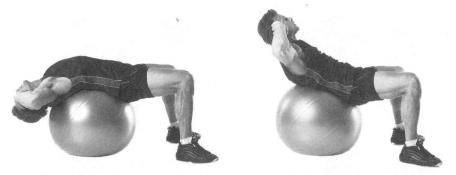

▶ Lie on your back on a Swiss ball, with both feet on the floor, just wider than shoulder-width apart. Your head should be slightly lower than your chest. Place your hands behind your ears, and point your elbows out.

▶ Curl your rib cage toward your pelvis while keeping your head and neck still.

▶ Hold, then return to the starting position.

▶ *If you're a beginner:* Place your hands on your chest, instead of behind your ears.

WORKOUT 2

Leg Press

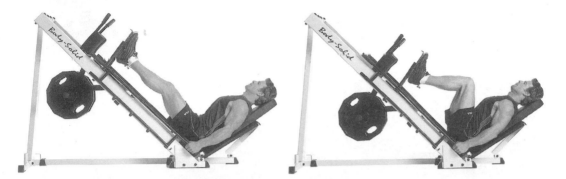

▶ Position yourself in the leg-press machine with your feet slightly wider than shoulder-width apart and toward the top of the platform. (Use the position that's most comfortable for your knees.) Straighten your legs without locking your knees.

▶ Release the supports, then lower the platform until your knees are bent 90 degrees. Keep your lower back against the pad throughout the movement.

▶ Push the platform back to the starting position.

▶ *If you're a beginner:* Use a very light weight and do the exercise as described.

Wide-Grip Barbell Bench Press

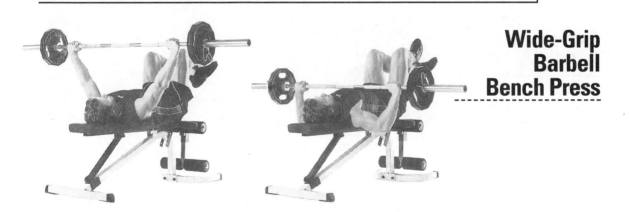

▶ Lie on your back on a flat bench with your legs raised up off the bench. Bend your hips and knees; cross your feet if you want. Grab the bar with an overhand grip, your hands a bit farther apart than for a standard barbell bench press, and lift it off the uprights. Hold it over your chin at arm's length.

▶ Slowly lower the bar to your chest.

▶ Pause, then push the bar back up until your arms are straight and the bar is over your chin again.

▶ *If you're a beginner:* Use light dumbbells.

Good Morning

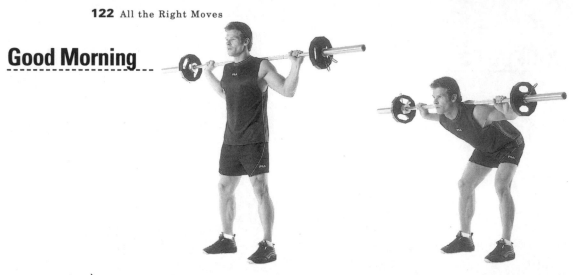

▶ Stand holding a barbell evenly across your shoulders and upper back muscles. Place your feet shoulder-width apart. Bend your knees slightly. Keep your lower back in its natural alignment.

▶ Slowly bend forward at the hips until your upper torso is parallel to the floor. Keep your lower back straight throughout.

▶ Raise your torso back to the starting position.

▶ *If you're a beginner:* Instead of using a barbell, hold your hands behind your head. When you can do this for 15 repetitions, move up to a bar.

Towel Pulldown

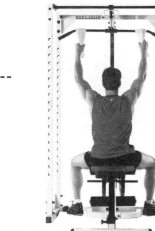
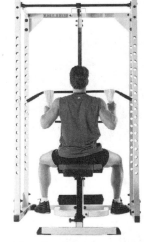

▶ Wrap a pair of towels around the bar of a lat-pulldown machine. Position yourself in the machine and grab a towel with each hand, keeping your hands just wider than shoulder-width apart.

▶ Pull the bar down to your chest as you lean backward slightly, keeping your back straight.

▶ Return to the starting position.

▶ *If you're a beginner:* Do a lat pulldown without the towels. Use an overhand grip that's just wider than your shoulders.

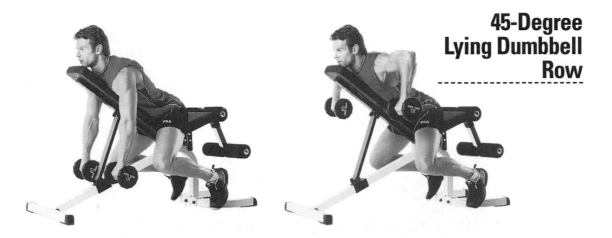

45-Degree Lying Dumbbell Row

▶ Set an incline bench to a 45-degree angle. Grab a pair of dumbbells and lie facedown on the bench, holding the weights straight down from your shoulders, with your palms turned toward your feet.

▶ Lift the weights up and out to your sides so your elbows are bent about 90 degrees and your upper arms are nearly perpendicular to your torso.

▶ Slowly return to the starting position.

▶ *If you're a beginner:* Do this exercise as described.

Towel Crunch

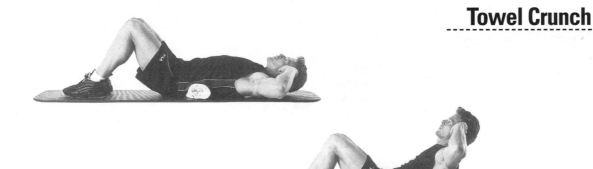

▶ Roll up a small towel and lie faceup with the towel in the arch of your lower back. Place your feet flat on the floor, put your hands behind your ears, and point your elbows out (not up).

▶ Curl your rib cage toward your pelvis, lifting your head and shoulders off the floor.

▶ Return to the starting position.

▶ *If you're a beginner:* Place your hands on your chest instead of behind your ears.

WORKOUT 3

Dumbbell Split Squat

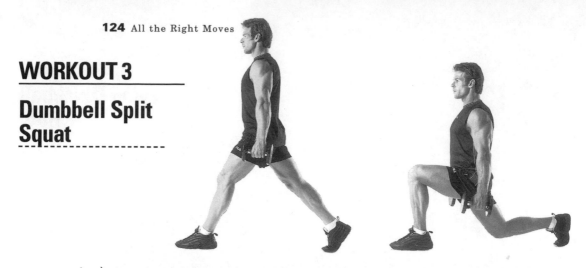

▶ Hold a pair of dumbbells at your sides as you stand with one foot about 3 feet in front of the other.

▶ Lower yourself until your front thigh is parallel to the floor and your rear knee almost touches the floor. (If your front lower leg is not perpendicular to the floor, start with a longer forward stride.)

▶ Return to the starting position and repeat for the designated number of reps. Then do the same number with your other leg forward.

▶ *If you're a beginner:* Hold your hands behind your head, rather than using dumbbells. When you can do all the reps in every set, do the exercise with weights.

Wide-Grip Stiff-Legged Deadlift

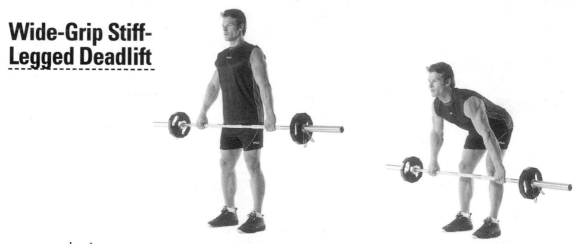

▶ Grab a barbell with an overhand grip that's about twice shoulder-width. Stand holding the bar down in front of you at arm's length and resting on your thighs. Set your feet shoulder-width apart, and bend your knees slightly. Keep your eyes focused straight ahead.

▶ Slowly bend at the hips as you lower the bar to just below your knees. During the move, do not bend your knees any more than they were bent in the starting position. Keep your head and chest up and your back straight.

▶ Lift your torso back to the starting position, keeping the bar as close to your body as possible.

▶ *If you're a beginner:* Do this exercise as described.

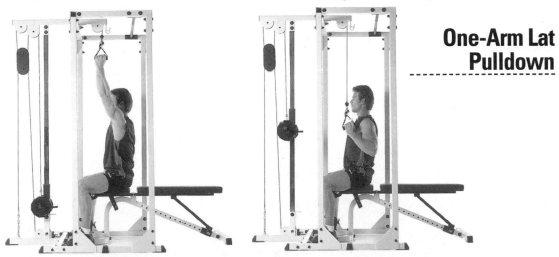

One-Arm Lat Pulldown

▶ Attach a stirrup handle to an overhead cable. Using an overhand grip, grab the handle with one hand (your left if you're right-handed) and position yourself in the machine with your working arm straight and the other down at your side.

▶ Pull the handle straight down until it's just outside your chest.

▶ Return to the starting position and repeat for the designated number of reps. Then do the same number with the other arm.

▶ *If you're a beginner:* Do the exercise as described.

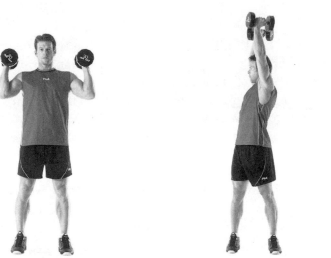

Twisting Dumbbell Shoulder Press

▶ Stand holding a pair of dumbbells at the sides of your shoulders, palms turned toward each other, feet shoulder-width apart, knees slightly bent, and lower back in its natural alignment.

▶ Lift the dumbbells straight over your shoulders as you twist your torso to the right.

▶ Lower the weights as you twist back to the starting position, then repeat to your left.

▶ *If you're a beginner:* Without twisting, lift the weights overhead one at a time.

Bridge

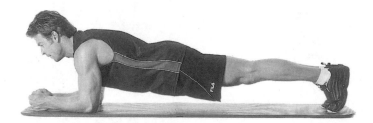

▶ Get into the pushup position on the floor with your weight resting on your forearms and toes, your back straight, and your head in line with your back. (You should be able to draw a straight line from your neck to your heels.) Look down at the floor.

▶ Pull in your abdomen as far as you can—imagine that you're trying to touch your belly button to your spine.

▶ Breathe as you hold in your abs for 10 seconds.

▶ Release and rest for a few seconds. Try to do a total of 6 repetitions.

▶ *If you're a beginner:* Try to do a total of 3 reps, building up to 6 reps.

CARDIOVASCULAR EXERCISE FOR WEIGHT LIFTERS

Ballantyne is very skeptical of the idea that hours and hours of endurance exercise are necessary to lose weight—especially if you're a big, fast-twitch-fiber guy. Sure, prolonged daily mileage burns a lot of calories. It also wears out your knees and uses your muscle tissue as an energy source.

A much better plan, in Ballantyne's view, is to spend the bulk of your exercise time and energy in the weight room, adding muscle, speeding up your metabolism, and making your body stronger and leaner instead of just smaller. Though the weights do

most of the work to transform your body, you can burn off some additional fat—without compromising your strength and muscle gains—by adding a type of aerobic exercise that Ballantyne calls *the new cardio*.

Others call it interval training, but Ballantyne likes to make a distinction: Interval training is usually an adjunct to long, slow, steady, aerobic exercise; whereas the new cardio is a replacement for long, slow, steady aerobics.

The new cardio works more like weight lifting. You go hard for a short period (usually 15 to 60 seconds), then easy for a minute or two.

Here's how to do it: Choose any

type of aerobic exercise you want—running, cycling, rowing. You can do it on a machine or the open road (or open river, if you're rowing). Then:

▶ Warm up for 5 minutes by going at a very easy pace, gradually increasing the effort until you're at about 50 percent of what you consider your maximum effort.

▶ Go as hard as you can for 15 seconds. If you're on a machine, this can mean cranking up the resistance of the machine (taking a stationary bike from level two to level six, for example), or increasing the speed (from 80 to 100 rpm, perhaps). Or do a combination of both that forces you to work as hard as seems possible.

▶ Recover for 2 minutes, going back to the pace at which you finished your warmup.

▶ Start the next interval, and repeat for the suggested number of intervals.

▶ Cool down for 5 minutes. (After your last 2-minute recovery, go at an even easier pace for another 3 minutes so your cooldown totals 5 minutes.)

THE BELLY-OFF 8-WEEK NEW-CARDIO PROGRAM

Do the new cardio one to three times a week, according to the following schedule.

Workout 1 (optional): 3 to 5 intervals

Workout 2 (recommended): 6 to 10 intervals

Workout 3 (optional): 3 to 5 intervals

After the first week or two, try to extend the length of your intervals without extending your recovery periods. Shoot for an extra 20 seconds per interval in one workout. If that works, move up to 25 seconds per interval in your subsequent workout, then 30 seconds at full effort in your next workout. Continue to use 2-minute recoveries.

When you can do 30-second intervals for a full week's worth of workouts, start shortening your recovery periods. Go hard for 30 seconds, then recover for 90 seconds instead of 2 minutes, and work your way down to 60-second recovery periods in subsequent workouts.

If you do all that and you still aren't finished with the 8-week program, make the intervals longer again—45 seconds, then 1 minute. At that duration, maintain a two-to-one ratio of recovery time to interval length: Recover for 90 seconds after a 45-second interval, and for 2 minutes following a 1-minute interval. If you have progressed to a very advanced stage, you can also go one-to-one if you keep intervals to 30 seconds.

If you really, really want to do the old cardio, the best time for it is at the very beginning of an exercise program. As you'll see in the "Belly-Off Success Story" profiles throughout this book, most men who drop a lot of weight start out doing traditional endurance exercise. Ballantyne doesn't think it's necessary, but it certainly can't hurt, and it will probably help in the beginning.

Only as Old as He Feels

LIFE IN THE FAT LANE

After an 8-year hitch in the U.S. Navy, Mike Brown returned to civilian life at a trim 160 pounds.

His new desk job, however, took its toll. By age 30, he weighed 215 pounds and looked like a stuffed sausage in his size-38 jeans.

Life was a Homer Simpson banquet: bacon-egg-and-cheese sandwiches for breakfast, doughnuts for a mid-morning snack, fried chicken or some chili dogs for lunch, whatever he wanted for dinner, and three or four beers a night.

He also smoked cigarettes—up to a pack a day.

Brown's vital signs suggested that he wouldn't live to a ripe old age. His blood pressure and cholesterol levels were elevated, he had a racing pulse, and he suffered chronic pain in his knees and lower back.

His scariest symptom was waking in the middle of the night due to acid reflux and not being able to breathe.

His doctor diagnosed him with a duodenal ulcer, placed him on medication, and instructed him to sleep with his head elevated.

THE TURNING POINT

Brown's ulcer gnawed on his psyche as much as on his gut. He worried that he had grown old before his time.

Then came the kicker: With a wife and two children at home, he tried to buy additional life insurance. The insurance company turned him down because of his high cholesterol.

"It was about 290," says Brown. "That's when I decided I would start shaping up."

THE PLAN OF ATTACK

For 3 months, he was the anti-Homer, eating fat-free yogurt with a banana and a glass of orange juice for breakfast, a turkey sandwich and a can of V8 for lunch, and either a soup-and-salad combo or a tuna sandwich for dinner. He also quit drinking beer.

For exercise, he began riding a bicycle every morning before work—until winter weather chased him back indoors. So he bought an exercise bike.

Soon, his morning regimen consisted of a strenuous 30 minutes on the bike, plus 25 pushups and 50 to 60 situps.

"After 3 or 4 months, I lost 55 pounds," he says. Almost before he knew it, he was wearing size-36 jeans, then size-34.

This was just the beginning. Brown scoured the Internet for advice that would not only keep him lean but also make him cut.

Name: MIKE BROWN
Date of Birth: March 1963
Occupation: Marine-supplies salesman
Height: 5 foot 9

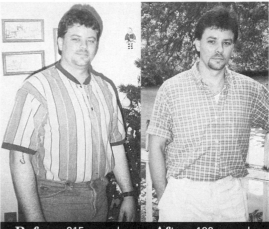

Before: 215 pounds   **After:** 180 pounds

He even bought a home gym, then traded it for a more expensive machine.

When even that failed to give him the desired results, he began training 3 days a week with dumbbells and an incline bench, followed by six abdominal exercises totaling 300 repetitions. He alternated those workouts with 3 days a week of cardiovascular exercise: 45 minutes on the stationary bike followed by 15 minutes on a treadmill.

60 min

Gradually, he began feeling the way nature intended a guy in his 30s to feel. Although he still needed medication to control his cholesterol, his blood pressure returned to normal, his knee and back pain disappeared, and his racing pulse slowed to a jog of 50 beats per minute. Even his ulcer cleared up, so he had no more scary acid-reflux episodes.

LIFE IN THE FIT LANE

By early 2001, Brown had reached a level of fitness that's a fantasy to many overweight guys. Still, he knew he could do even better. "I was still trying to burn off that last bit of fat, so my goals changed," he says.

He switched to a more traditional bodybuilding diet: high protein, medium carbohydrate, and low fat. Today, he eats oatmeal and eggs for breakfast, a sandwich for a snack, and tuna and salad for lunch.

"I've been eating more good food," he says. "Right now, I probably take in around 2,700 to 3,000 calories a day."

Although he's gained back some weight, almost all of it is lean tissue. He still wears size-34 jeans.

Brown's home exercise program also has undergone a drastic overhaul. He still has his trusty exercise bike, but he uses it only for a 5-to-7-minute warmup. Then he stretches for 15 minutes and starts his lifting routine. "I don't do as much cardio as I used to," he says. "Weight lifting is the better way to go."

He lifts on Sundays, Tuesdays, and Thursdays for about an hour, training different body parts each day.

Brown super-sizes his results by taking creatine before his workouts and drinking a protein shake afterward. The results of the workouts and supplements are so good that he's begun dispensing advice on Internet forums.

Among his tips is the following recipe for a post-workout shake that provides a 3-to-1 ratio of carbs to protein: one banana, one 28-gram scoop of dextrose (a sweetener you can purchase in bulk at health food stores or through www.proteinfactory.com), one 28-gram scoop of strawberry whey protein powder, 12 ounces of water, and a handful of ice.

Brown's efforts left him with a single vestige of the bad old days: his smoking habit. In March 2001, he began taking the antidepressant Wellbutrin SR (bupropion hydrochloride)— commonly used in smoking-cessation programs. After 2 weeks on the drug, he was able to kick his cigarette habit.

"It was a piece of cake," Brown says.

HIS TIPS

REST IS KEY. "Overtraining can hinder any gains, cause injury, and discourage you from your goals. Since you actually build size while you're resting, I also try to get 8 hours of sleep a night."

TAKE A DAY OFF. "Don't forget to reward yourself with one cheat day a week for all the hard work and effort you put in to make yourself feel and look your best."

CHAPTER
12

The Benefits of
Aerobic Exercise

COMPARED WITH WEIGHT TRAINING, AEROBIC EXERCISE HAS BEEN oversold to the American public. Not that aerobic exercise isn't healthful or beneficial. If it were of no value, it wouldn't have been emphasized in the first place, much less overemphasized. Among the benefits:

▶ Decreased fat, especially visceral fat

▶ Increased bone strength beneath the muscles used in the activity (hips and legs for runners, upper body for swimmers, etcetera)

▶ Improved immune-system function

▶ Increased HDL ("good") cholesterol

▶ Lower resting heart rate

▶ Lower blood pressure

▶ Improved insulin sensitivity

If aerobic exercise were the only way to get all these benefits, as scientists believed until recently, we would unequivocally advocate it over strength training. Research has shown, however, that all these benefits can be derived with a combination of strength training and diet. That brings up a very good question: What benefits does aerobic exercise provide that you can't get by any other means?

One thing: increased aerobic power, which researchers call VO_2 max, or maximal oxygen uptake. Anybody can improve his aerobic power, of course, but as with everything else in life, some people are born with a genetic advantage. A 1999 study in the *Journal of Applied Physiology* found that VO_2 max is about 59 percent inherited. The VO_2 max response to exercise—how much you improve once you start working out—is about 47 percent genetic.

Here's why this is important for a guy who wants to lose weight: When you're completely out of shape and you start exercising, it takes a long time before you can work long enough and intensely enough to burn a lot of calories and achieve noticeable weight loss. But if you're genetically programmed to have greater aerobic fitness, you'll be able to burn a significant number of calories—and thus see results—sooner. On top of that, you'll likely enjoy the exercise more. After all, who doesn't prefer to do what he knows he can do well? (Golfers, perhaps, but that's a different book.)

So one argument in favor of aerobic exercise is that some people are

Belly Busters

▶▶ "My idea of exercise used to be just making it up the stairs or going around the block. Now I walk approximately 1½ hours a day and use my stationary bike for about 1 hour a day with no difficulty at all.

"The program we tried worked for both my wife and me. We lost a total of 204½ pounds. We may not live longer, but I can assure you that we can enjoy ourselves 100 percent more." ◀◀

—DON FITZGERALD
67, LOST 153 POUNDS

genetically programmed to be good at it. (These people include not only those with a VO_2 max advantage but also, as mentioned in the previous chapter, those with a higher proportion of slow-twitch muscle fibers.) If they perform aerobic activities, genetics may allow them to do so longer and harder—and see results faster—than people without that propensity.

For those who aren't genetically gifted that way, the best reason to do aerobic exercise is that, while harder is better than easier, even a minimal amount does produce some health benefits. For example, an Oklahoma State University study surveyed absentee records of 79,000 employees and found that those who did aerobic exercise for just 20 minutes, twice a week, took fewer sick days than those who didn't exercise at all.

Another argument for the aerobically gifted and nongifted alike is that a guy with a higher level of cardiovascular fitness burns a higher proportion of fat calories at rest and during most other activities. (In all-out activities, he still burns mostly carbohydrates for energy.) That doesn't mean he burns more total calories over the course of the day—that would imply a higher resting metabolism, and most studies show endurance exercise won't increase your metabolism when you aren't exercising. It just means that he's more likely to use his body's fat for energy.

AEROBICS VERSUS WEIGHTS

So there we have a series of reasonably compelling reasons for a guy to take up aerobic exercise or, if he already does it and enjoys it, to continue it. The problem is the notion that everyone has to do some form of aerobic exercise, no matter his goals, interests, condition, or genetic predisposition.

In fact, strength training may be far more beneficial to far more people than traditional aerobic exercise, because improved VO_2 max means very little to the average guy. There are three reasons for this.

1. Weight training may not improve VO_2 max, but it doesn't lower it below baseline levels either. In other words, guys who lift weights exclusively don't *lose* any aerobic fitness. That only happens if you quit exercising altogether. (For someone with below-normal VO_2

max, you can probably make a stronger argument for aerobic exercise—or simply for weight loss. VO_2 max is a calculation based on body mass, so if you have a smaller body, your aerobic fitness automatically improves. Losing 20 pounds, for example, could improve your VO_2 max by 10 percent.)

2. Even though weight training doesn't do much to improve VO_2 max, it does improve a person's endurance *performance* as measured by maximum time to exhaustion on a treadmill test. Apparently, the strength of the specific muscles necessary for doing an activity is a key factor in how long you can do it without stopping to rest. This leads to a pretty good question: If both aerobic exercise and weight training produce the same result—you can do more work before you get exhausted—what difference does it make that one form of exercise improves VO_2 max and the other doesn't?

3. The only sports in which VO_2 max is an important factor in performance are the obvious ones: long-distance endurance sports such as running and cycling, and heavy-endurance team sports such as soccer. (Even in those, fitness markers such as lactate threshold may be more crucial to success.) You don't have to increase your VO_2 max to become a better football or basketball player, although it may help. Most sports involve rapid starts, stops, and changes of direction, and endurance training doesn't prepare you for those moves any better than reading this sentence does.

Here's another way to look at the cardio-versus-weights issue: If you argue that VO$_2$ max is meaningless, you should be able to prove that the one unique benefit of weight training—increased muscle mass and strength—is meaningful.

If you look at a 50-year-old guy who's never lifted weights, you see someone who within 10 years will probably lose 12 to 14 percent of his strength, along with 6 percent of his muscle mass. Those losses put him at risk for increased falls, hip fractures, glucose intolerance, and any number of diseases and disabilities. Just 2 months of strength training can reverse 2 decades of strength and muscle loss, and no gain in VO$_2$ max could have that effect. This seems pretty meaningful.

Yet, say you have a 25-year-old guy who adds an inch to his arms or 50 pounds to his maximum bench press. Has he done anything to extend his life or improve his health? Sure, if he's made these gains without appreciably expanding his waistline. But lots of young guys eat anything and everything to get those 17-inch arms or a 300-pound max bench press. A guy who adds 4 inches of fat to his waist while adding 1 inch of muscle to his arms is most likely compromising his health rather than meaningfully improving it.

Research shows that you aren't going to achieve great results with ei-

Belly Busters

▶▶ "I began walking every night. I started with short walks through the neighborhood, then began making them longer. One day, while walking, I decided, 'Maybe I can jog to that light post down there.' Each day, I would make my jogging periods longer. Soon, I was running the entire route." ◀◀

—STEVEN KLAPOW
32, LOST 57 POUNDS

ther form of exercise if you don't also modify your diet, and you probably aren't going to achieve lasting weight loss if you make dietary modifications without doing either weight training or aerobic exercise.

So it seems clear that, depending on your genetics, both forms of exercise can be used to achieve better health, a longer life, and a leaner waist.

Thus, let's declare a cease-fire in the war between cardio guys and muscleheads. Everybody's right, since some exercise is better than none; and nobody's wrong, since doing the exercise you prefer is far more likely to bring you benefits than pursuing a form of fitness you feel your body is resisting.

Now let's look at how someone who wants to pursue aerobic exercise can get those benefits.

AEROBICS FOR WEIGHT LOSS

When you're trying to lose weight, there's a huge strategic difference between cardiovascular exercise and weight training. With strength exercise, you want to build up to the point where you can lift intensely for about 45 minutes three or four times a week. Strength training does its work in between sessions, when your chronically elevated metabolism chips away at your belly fat. You can lift more often if you have a specific reason for doing so and a program designed for that many days of lifting. But if you're doing a program created for average guys—such as the one in this book—too much training can compromise your strength and muscle gains and interrupt this metabolic mechanism.

Cardiovascular exercise is different. You want to increase your exercise volume gradually until you're training for at least 30 minutes almost every day of the week. You need near-daily exercise to burn off enough calories to make a difference. Plus, aerobic exercise elevates your metabolism only while you're doing it and for a short

time—perhaps an hour or two—afterward.

The key word in the previous paragraph is *gradually*, for two reasons. First, if you don't start slowly, your aching muscles will tell you about it the next day—and nothing saps your motivation like excessive pain and stiffness. Second, a slow start and gradual buildup gives your connective tissues a chance to adapt to the exercise, heading off long-term overuse injuries such as tendonitis, bursitis, and lots of other conditions. Your muscles and lungs may seem ready for major leaps in exercise volume after the first couple weeks, but your connective tissues probably aren't prepared. Your tendons and ligaments have fewer blood vessels than your muscles, so they make slower adaptations to exercise. They also take longer to recover from injuries.

Walking is probably the safest and easiest form of aerobic exercise. Ultimately, it doesn't matter which you choose—cycling, swimming, rowing, inline dogsledding. You'll get the most benefit from the one you enjoy the most and pursue the most deliberately.

One caveat: We don't recommend jogging or running for heavier guys. If you're more than 15 pounds over your fighting weight, lose weight first, jog second. Running is just flat-out tough on your knees, and the more you weigh, the more impact your knees have to absorb. Runner's knee is the number one chronic sports injury in

Belly Busters

▶▶ "I started walking every day. I reached the point where I could walk over 5 miles per workout. When that happened, I started to jog. I started slow jogging for only a mile. Each week, I would add ¹⁄₁₀ mile. I worked myself up to the 3 miles that I now jog. I listen to fast-paced music to keep me going." ◀◀

—REY SIFUENTES JR.
28, LOST 91 POUNDS

America, according to the Cooper Institute for Aerobics Research. This despite the fact that running is only the fifth-most-popular exercise.

THE BELLY-OFF 8-WEEK AEROBIC-EXERCISE PROGRAM

The table below provides a sample aerobic-exercise schedule for someone who hasn't exercised regularly in recent memory. The first three columns are self-explanatory, but "% of Full Effort" can be interpreted a few different ways. One is to look at it as a percentage of your maximum heart rate, or MHR. That maximum is usually described as "220 minus your age," so if you're 40, your MHR would be 180 beats per minute. Sixty percent of your maximum is 106, and 70 percent is 126.

There's an unfortunate problem with this method: Maximum heart rate, like VO_2 max, is for the most part genetically determined. Only a slim majority of the population has an exact 220-minus-age MHR. For the rest of us, MHR can vary by as much

Aerobic-Exercise Schedule

Week	Days	Minutes	% of Full Effort
1	3	10	60
2	3	15	60
3	4	15	65
4	4	20	65
5	4	20	70
6	4	25	70
7	5	25	70
8	5	30	70

as 60 beats per minute. The older you are, the less likely you'll be close to the MHR determined by this method. A 40-year-old guy could have an actual MHR of anywhere from 150 to 210 beats per minute.

Another way to gauge effort is *perceived exertion,* or how hard exercise feels at the time you're doing it. At 55-percent exertion, you start to feel that you're exercising and starting to move a little faster, as opposed to strolling along as you enjoy the scenery. You can still talk normally and breathe comfortably.

At 75 percent of top effort, your breathing is deeper but remains steady. This feels like exercise, beyond any doubt, and starts to feel like *hard* exercise. You can still exchange snatches of conversation, but only in short sentences and only if the woman you're talking to is exceptionally attractive.

So you'll want to keep your efforts between these two extremes.

Finally, before each workout, make sure to warm up for 5 minutes at 40 to 50 percent of maximum effort. Cool down afterward for 5 minutes at the same pace as your warmup. The 10-minute workouts in the first week are really 20 minutes, counting warmups and cooldowns. And the 30-minute workouts in week 8 are 40 minutes total.

MIXING IT UP

Once you get past this break-in program, you'll probably want to add some new-cardio workouts, as de-

Belly Busters

▶▶ "A couple of years ago, I wanted to shed an inch or two from my waist and have my pants fit better. I tried different exercises, with no results. I talked to a coworker who was also an aerobics instructor, and she recommended buying and using a heart-rate monitor to make sure I was staying in my target zone. I bought one and used it regularly, and was able to track my progress. After a few months, my pants began to fit better." ◀◀

—TOM SCHOLTEN
33, LOST 10 POUNDS

scribed in the previous chapter. For one thing, interval training makes your workouts more interesting. Instead of zoning out, you truly focus on what you're doing. You'll also get through your workout faster—perhaps in 25 minutes instead of 40—and the time will pass much more quickly.

You'll also burn much more fat with intervals than with steady-pace endurance exercise. Many studies have shown this, but one of the first was conducted by Canadian researchers and published in *Metabolism* in 1994. In that one, study subjects were divided into two groups: One did traditional steady-pace endurance exercise for 20 weeks, working up to 30 to 45 minutes 4 or 5 days a week. The second group did the new cardio: high-intensity intervals of either 15 to 30 seconds or 60 to 90 seconds, with full recovery in between intervals, meaning they allowed their heart rates to return to 120 to 130 beats per min-

utes. (The exercisers were 18 to 32 years old, so that heart rate represents a fairly light level of exertion.)

At the end of the study, the researchers estimated that the first group, doing traditional endurance exercise, had expended twice as many calories as the second group. Yet the second group lost more subcutaneous fat. "Moreover, when the difference in the total energy cost of the two programs was taken into account . . . the subcutaneous fat loss was ninefold greater" in the interval program than in the traditional endurance program, the researchers concluded.

This demonstrates the power of the "afterburn," or the increased use of fat for energy that occurs after an interval workout. (You get the same effect following heavier strength training.) You don't get this effect from long, steady-pace endurance exercise, although you use fat for energy *during* that more traditional type of aerobic workout.

Here's a sample aerobic-training schedule utilizing both traditional endurance exercise and the new cardio.

Sunday: Steady pace for 50 to 60 minutes

Monday: Rest

Tuesday: New cardio for 20 minutes

Wednesday: Steady pace for 20 to 30 minutes

Thursday: Rest

Friday: New cardio for 20 to 30 minutes

Saturday: Steady pace for 30 to 40 minutes

Remember to add 5 minutes to the beginning and end of each workout for warmup and cooldown.

WEIGHT TRAINING FOR CARDIO GUYS

Most forms of aerobic exercise overwork one set of muscles and underwork another. A runner, to pick the most obvious example, ends up with very tight muscles on the back of his body—calves, hamstrings, gluteals, lower back—and relatively weak muscles on the front. Many sports-medicine physicians and physical therapists believe this imbalance leads to knee injuries, as the tighter muscles pull the kneecaps out of their natural position and aggravate the knees' connective tissues. At the same time, posture is important for a runner: He has to hold himself upright over long distances to be able to perform well.

So an ideal strength-training program for walkers, joggers, or runners would include these five exercises, shown in the previous chapter.

- ▶ Barbell squat
- ▶ Wide-grip seated row
- ▶ Wide-grip barbell bench press
- ▶ Towel crunch
- ▶ Wide-grip stiff-legged deadlift

Start with 1 set of 20 repetitions of each of these exercises, two times a week. (Do them before your aerobic workouts, if that's possible. In the schedule shown on the previous page, these workouts would go well with the new-cardio sessions on Tuesday and Friday.)

After 2 weeks, increase the amount of weight you use and decrease repetitions so you do 1 set of 12 to 15 repetitions.

After another 2 weeks, increase the weight again and decrease repetitions so you do 2 or 3 sets of 10 reps.

For the 7th and 8th weeks, increase the weight again and do 3 or 4 sets of 8 repetitions.

After the 8th week, switch exercises, choosing others from the previous chapter, or from *Men's Health* magazine or another impeccable source.

Cop Arrests Diabetes

LIFE IN THE FAT LANE

William Senik was a trim 177 pounds when he graduated from the New York State Police Academy at age 27. During his first few years on the beat, he stayed trim, contradicting the stereotype about big cops and big doughnuts.

Then he was promoted to sergeant and found himself spending more time behind a desk. Along the way, he also got married and had a son. "The pounds just crept up," he says.

In January 2000, he jumped at the chance to become a plain-clothes investigator. But he found a disturbing link between "undercover" and "overweight." "I had to eat most of my meals on the run, and my diet was atrocious," he says. A typical lunch was a Whopper, french fries, and a Coke. For dinner, he ate lots of juicy steaks and fried foods.

In spite of his eating habits, a physical in the summer of 2000 showed that his cholesterol and blood sugar were normal. Still,

Senik knew that he needed to lose weight. At 212 pounds, he couldn't climb the four flights of stairs to his office without getting winded.

It was only a matter of time, he says, before his superiors would have put him on the "fat-boy list." "We have a height/weight requirement, and if you don't fall into that, you have to correct it."

It turned out that the possibility of landing on the list was the least of his problems.

THE TURNING POINT

In early 2001, Senik suddenly had difficulty reading license plates and street addresses while doing surveillance.

He had other troubling symptoms, including an unquenchable thirst and a frequent need to urinate. At work, his partner kidded him about constantly needing to "take a personal."

His family doctor confirmed

that his blood-glucose level was 420. He had type-2, or adult-onset, diabetes.

"I was crushed," he says. "I thought I had been handed a death sentence. But my doctor assured me all was not lost."

THE PLAN OF ATTACK

To lower his blood sugar, Senik's doctor gave him an insulin shot, then put him on two oral medications. The doc also issued some stern advice: Eat right, exercise more, and lose 35 pounds.

"I was determined this disease would not beat me," says Senik.

Name: WILLIAM SENIK
Date of Birth: March 1960
Residence: Peekskill, New York
Occupation: Investigator, New York State Police
Height: 5 foot 10

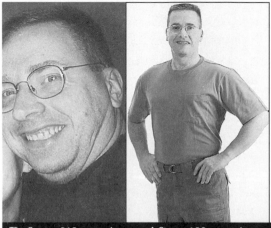

Before: 212 pounds   **After:** 180 pounds

He learned more about diabetes and its complications, including a fluid buildup in the eyes that causes deteriorating vision and, in extreme cases, blindness. He also learned to inspect food labels for grams of carbohydrates and fats.

"My eating habits changed dramatically," he says. "I reduced my carbohydrate intake to less than 125 grams a day."

He switched from red meat to chicken and turkey, and from starchy foods to broccoli, string beans, and other vegetables. Instead of three big meals a day, he ate three smaller meals, plus snacks. His meals included a bowl of high-fiber cereal for breakfast; a graham cracker or nuts for a mid-morning snack; and brown-bag lunches consisting of turkey chili or a tuna sandwich with low-fat mayo on 12-grain bread. He used a hand-held-computer program called Eat It to track his carbohydrate consumption and weight loss.

Senik also dramatically increased his exercise intensity. "I began walking and running on a treadmill for a minimum of one half-hour a day, every day," he says. "On alternate days, I focused on my circuit training,

which included 11 different workstations, doing 3 sets on each piece of equipment."

By April 2001, Senik's blood-sugar levels had declined so much that his doctor told him to stop taking his diabetes medications.

"I was actually a little fearful," he says. "I didn't know if I could do it on my own." After several weeks, however, he realized he could control his blood sugar naturally. That bolstered his self-confidence and his determination to stick with his new lifestyle.

By July 2001, Senik had lost 32 pounds, which put him just 3 pounds short of his goal. His belly was flat. In just 5 months, he had gone from a "real tight size-36" to a "real loose size-33."

LIFE IN THE FIT LANE

No longer does Senik find it taxing to climb four flights of stairs. No longer does he have to take so many "personals" at work or in the middle of the night. Even his blurry vision has cleared up.

He now runs 2 to 3 miles three or four times a week, even if he has to do so at odd hours. When he can't run outdoors, he runs on a home treadmill. "The amount of weight I lift has gone up exponentially."

He measures his blood sugar twice a day, and he has learned to read his body: If his blood sugar is too low, he feels edgy. If it's too high, he feels fatigued.

HIS TIPS FOR DIABETICS

STAY VIGILANT. "Never forget, this disease doesn't go away. There is no cure yet. If you let this get away from you, it could kill you."

AVOID SELF-PITY. "Granted, every situation with diabetes is different, but never allow yourself to become a victim. Do whatever you have to do. Your life depends on it."

DRINK SAFELY. "If you have diabetes, you have to be careful because alcohol lowers your blood sugar. If you have a couple of beers, you have to eat a little something, maybe even something a little starchy." *Note:* If your diabetes is under control and you've been given the green light by your doctor, it's okay to drink in moderation. That means no more than two drinks a day for a man, according to the American Diabetes Association. As Senik notes, you should *never* drink alcohol on an empty stomach. Plan to have your drink with a meal or after eating a snack.

May 2006.

Keeping Your Body Loose and Ready for Use

ACCORDING TO THE SPORTING GOODS MANUFACTURING ASSOCIATION, 13.7 million men used stretching as a fitness activity in 2000 (along with 22.7 million women). Almost 7 million men stretched at least 100 times that year. The only fitness activity that more men did as frequently was weight lifting (9.3 million). By contrast, 5.5 million men ran or jogged at least 100 times, and 6.4 million walked for exercise.

Apparently, guys would rather feel limber and athletic than stiff and creaky. Shocking, huh?

Okay, not really. But here's something that may come as a surprise.

For years, guys have been told that they should stretch as a warmup because it prevents injuries. You've heard that plenty of times, right? But Canadian researcher Ian Shrier, M.D., Ph.D., reviewed the existing research and declared there's no evidence for this belief.

Sure, a warmup prevents injuries. But it doesn't seem to matter whether or not that warmup includes formal stretching.

Another assumption was that stretching has some sort of permanent effect on the stiffness or length of muscles and tendons (the connective tissues that attach muscles to bones). This doesn't seem to be true, either. Most likely, muscles and connective tissues simply develop a tolerance for the pain of stretching. "Range of motion in humans might be primarily limited by pain," Dr. Shrier and coauthor Kav Gossal, M.D., wrote in *The Physician and Sportsmedicine*.

HOW AND WHY TO STRETCH

Despite puncturing a few beliefs about what stretching is and what it can do for your body, Dr. Shrier never suggests it's a waste of time. Rather, he shows that what we don't know about stretching far outpaces what we do know.

Still, we bet you'd appreciate some general advice on limbering up, so here goes.

How long: Lots of researchers have tried to offer a guideline, and Dr. Shrier concludes that a stretch held for about 30 seconds offers the most benefit in the least time. Some muscles may need a longer stretch, and some may do better with a shorter one: The 30-second recommendation is just an average. If your hamstrings don't seem to loosen up in 30 seconds, try 45. For some upper-body muscles, a 10-second stretch may feel as good as 30 seconds.

How: Dr. Shrier prefers the technique advocated by Bob Anderson in

the book *Stretching*: Stretch a muscle until you feel some tension or a slight pulling sensation, but not pain. Hold that position until you feel the muscle relax, then stretch it a bit farther until you feel the tension again. Hold that stretch until you feel the muscle relax again. Try stretching it again but stop when you can't stretch any farther. In other words, let your muscles tell you how far to stretch.

When: Like any other form of exercise, stretching seems to work best if you do it when you want to and when you can.

You may have heard the warning that you should never stretch a cold muscle. It's true that a cold muscle won't stretch as far as a warm one. That doesn't mean you have to go through an elaborate warmup ritual every time you feel like stretching. If you follow the "How" recommendation above, you'll never hurt yourself stretching. You'll simply stretch the muscle until you feel some tension, wait for the tension to relax, then stretch it a little farther until you feel more tension.

On the other hand, you can easily injure a fully warmed-up muscle by stretching it farther than it wants to go—taking it past the point of mild tension into the realm of pain.

The key, as mentioned above: Never stretch your muscles farther than they want to go. Some days they'll stretch farther than others. Still other days, your limbs will feel mummified. Pay attention to your muscles, and you'll get all the benefits of stretching with no chance of injury.

STRETCHING FOR WEIGHT LOSS?

Sorry. An average 200-pound guy would burn only 200 calories stretching for an hour. That's just 64 more calories than he would burn sitting and watching someone else stretch. Ignoring for a moment the fact that no guy is going to stretch for an hour, the impact of 64 calories on a 200-pound man is, frankly, negligible. That doesn't mean 5 to 10 minutes of stretching before a workout will have a negligible effect on a guy's waistline. If it helps him enjoy his workout more and makes the exercises seem more productive, it's worthwhile.

Consider this: With 45 minutes of high-intensity weight lifting, this same 200-pounder can burn more than 400 calories, which is really just a prelude to all the metabolic benefits described in chapter 11. In 30 minutes of moderate pedaling on a stationary bike, he can burn 319 calories.

If those 5 to 10 minutes of stretching allow him to do those workouts more often and more successfully, they do indeed help him lose his gut.

But stretching by itself is extremely unlikely to take inches off your waist.

A FEW GOOD STRETCHES

Here's a nice series of general stretches that most guys should be able to do. You can do them before or after a workout, or at any other time of day. Try holding each stretch for 10 seconds at first, then progress to 30 seconds on the lower-body stretches and perhaps 15 to 20 seconds on the upper-body moves. (If 10 seconds feels as if it does the trick for your shoulders or neck, don't feel obligated to hold the stretches longer.)

Your back, neck, and shoulders should feel better within weeks, if not days.

UPPER BODY

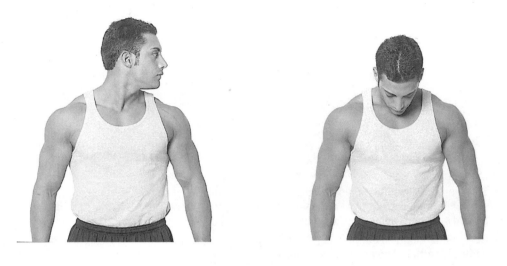

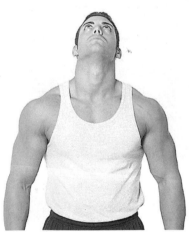

▶ Stand with your back straight and your legs shoulder-width apart. Your neck should be straight and your shoulders relaxed.

▶ Slowly turn your head to the right as far as it will comfortably go. Hold for 10 seconds. Repeat to the left. Return to the starting position.

▶ Without bending your upper body, tuck your chin into your chest until you feel a mild pull in the back of your neck. Hold for 10 seconds.

▶ Slowly tilt your head back until you're looking straight up, but not so far back that your head rests on your shoulders. Hold for 10 seconds, then relax.

Overhead Shoulder Stretch

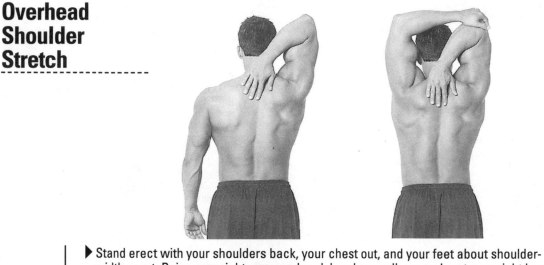

▶ Stand erect with your shoulders back, your chest out, and your feet about shoulder-width apart. Raise your right arm overhead, bend your elbow, and rest your right hand behind your neck, just between your shoulder blades.

▶ Use your left hand to gently push on your right elbow, edging it toward the center of your body and farther down behind your neck.

▶ Switch arms and repeat.

Chest Stretch

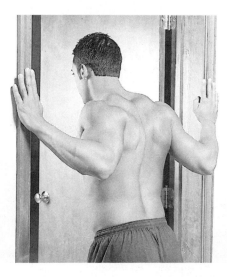

▶ Place your hands on both sides of a doorway at shoulder height. Keep your chest and head up and your knees slightly bent.

▶ Move your upper body forward until you feel a comfortable stretch. Hold the position for 10 seconds, but do not hold your breath. Do once.

LOWER BODY

Spinal Twist

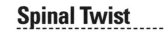
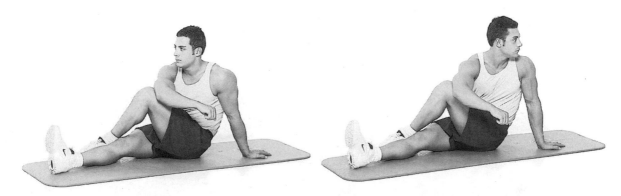

▶ Sit on the floor with both legs extended. Bend your left leg over your right, placing your left foot flat on the floor outside your right knee. Place your right elbow on the outside of your left knee, and extend your left arm behind you with your palm flat on the floor for support.

▶ Twist your upper body to the left by slowly looking over your left shoulder. As you twist, press your right elbow against the outside of your left knee. Keep your upper body straight. Hold.

▶ Switch sides and repeat.

Lying Leg Pull

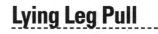
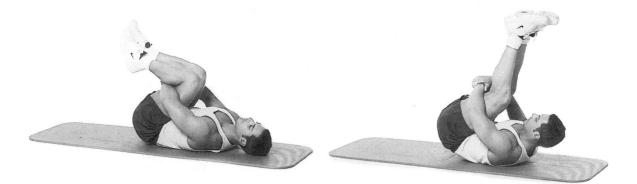

▶ Lie on your back. With your forearms under your thighs, pull your knees as close to your chest as they will comfortably go. This stretches your lower back.

▶ Keeping your knees close to your chest, extend your legs over your head. This extends the stretch to include your hamstrings and butt muscles. Hold for 10 seconds, then return to the starting position. Do once.

Butterfly Stretch
- - - - - - - - - - - - - - - - - - -

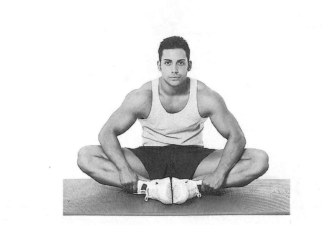

▶ Sit on the floor with your legs bent frog-style, the soles of your feet pressed together. Gently press your knees toward the floor with your elbows or hands. Hold.

Hamstring Stretch
- - - - - - - - - - - - - - - - - - -

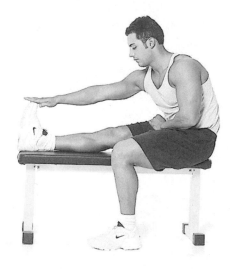

▶ Sit on the edge of a bench or bed with your right leg extended on it and your left foot on the floor. (This position takes stress off your lower back, unlike similar stretches in which you sit on the floor.) Rest your right hand on your right knee, then slowly slide your fingers to your toes, reaching as far as is comfortable. Hold.

▶ Switch legs and repeat.

Thigh Pull

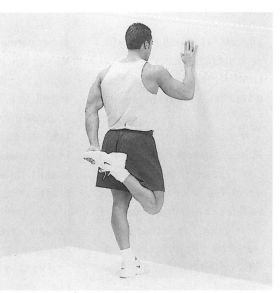

▶ Stand in front of a wall or chair, resting your right hand on it for support. Bend your right knee and grab that foot with your left hand, pulling your foot up so that your heel presses against your butt. Hold.

▶ Switch legs and repeat.

Calf Stretch

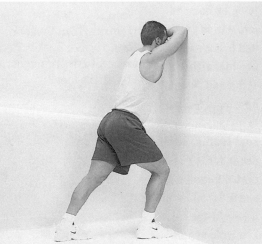

▶ Stand slightly away from a wall and lean on it with your forearms, your head on your hands. Place your right foot in front of you, leg bent. Your left leg should extend straight behind you.

▶ Slowly move your hips forward until you feel a stretch in your left calf. Keep your left heel flat and your toes pointed straight ahead. Hold an easy stretch for 10 seconds.

▶ Switch legs and repeat.

Grandfather Cause

LIFE IN THE FAT LANE

The owner of three businesses, Ki Martin passed his days in traffic or the office. This left little time for meals. Oh, Martin ate—just all the wrong things. "All I ate was fast food. McDonald's for breakfast, Burger King for lunch, and McDonald's for dinner," he says.

After 18 years of this, he weighed just over 300 pounds—enough to fill out size-48 pants. Not surprisingly, he also suffered chronic heartburn.

THE TURNING POINT

In 2000, Martin closed his businesses to help care for his sick grandmother. While working in his grandparents' backyard, he noticed an odd contraption hanging from a tree: two heavy stones fastened on either end of a rope, attached to a pulley. When he asked his granddad what it was, the older man grabbed it with one hand and did a pulldown—something nearly impossible for Martin himself. "I realized that my 95-year-old grandfather was healthier than I was," he admits. It was time to reassess his life.

THE PLAN OF ATTACK

Martin's first step was a literal one: "I began to walk down the street. The first day, I just went up three or four mailboxes and came back. The next day, I walked a little bit farther, and a little bit farther," he says. Next, he mixed in small amounts of jogging. "Within the first month, I dropped 6 or 7 pounds." He was still eating junk, but already he felt better.

About 3 months later, he bumped into a friend who had lost weight and looked great. "I thought, 'It must be a good feeling to be that fit,'" says Martin. So he asked for her secret. It turned out she was following a weight-loss plan involving supplement shakes. "I tried one and it was awful," he says. But the rest of her eating plan passed his muster when he realized it was simply a portion-controlled, balanced diet.

So Martin eighty-sixed fast food and began eating three healthy meals a day, plus two snacks. He also ditched all beverages other than water. "After about a month, I noticed that my clothes were getting loose. The first time I got on the scale to officially start charting, I was 289. I had probably dropped 15 pounds," he says.

Martin was a convert—and still is. For breakfast, he grabs a bagel with cappuccino spread.

Name: KI MARTIN
Occupation: Owner of a tree service
Residence: Ruskin, Florida
Date of Birth: August 1960
Height: 5 foot 8

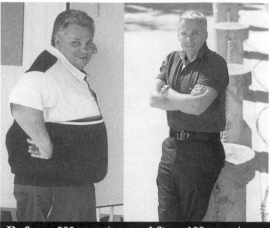

Before: 300 pounds   **After:** 168 pounds

Lunch is turkey and cheese on rye with tomato and a little mayo. Then he has two pieces of fruit. For dinner, Martin tosses back 4 to 6 ounces of chicken, fish, or turkey; with a grain, a vegetable, and a salad. He satisfies his sweet tooth with a dessert such as low-fat chocolate pudding. He snacks twice a day—typically fruit or rye-crisp crackers with butter and cheese. If he goes out to eat, he keeps portion control in mind.

After he had a handle on his eating and started feeling better, Martin's friend suggested he call her personal trainer. The first thing the trainer told him was, "You're going to have to lose weight *and* build strength to be a healthy person." This was news to Martin. "I thought that weight lifting is for guys who want to be bulky," he says. "It's not."

He spent weeks with the trainer, developing workouts for all the major muscle groups. Then he was on his own. "All of a sudden, I was dropping 3 pounds a week," he says. "Now the whole thing was working: I quit eating the food. I was drinking a lot of water. And the weight lifting." Within a year, he hit 161 pounds, with a 31-inch waist.

LIFE IN THE FIT LANE

Martin received a payload of benefits for his hard work. For starters, the heartburn disappeared. "I was eating Rolaids like M&M's. Now, if I want to go out at 10:00 at night and eat the spiciest chicken wings they make, I can go to sleep afterward," he says.

Martin swims in the clothes he once bought at the big-and-tall shop. "I would have never thought in my life that I was going to wear a size-medium shirt. Now I wear a small or medium," he says.

He's also become a much more active person. "I have twice the energy that I did before." He even started a new business cutting down trees. And he returned to a post he had held when he was much younger: volunteer firefighter.

Best of all? He can throw around stones with the best of them: his grandfather.

HIS WORKOUT

Martin alternates cardio with strength training. His cardio includes at least 3 days a week of running, walking, or cycling. As for muscle building, he bought a $267 home gym at a local dis-count store. He does 3 sets of 8 reps of the following exercises: bench presses, flies, rows, calf raises, squats, and crunches.

HIS TIPS

GET A SECOND OPINION. "I had gone in for a physical about 2 months before I started on this weight loss, and I said, 'I think I'm going to shave a little bit of weight. Do you have any recommendations?' The guy handed me the food-guide pyramid but didn't say a word about exercise."

DOWNSIZE PORTIONS. "The world is pretty much set up to hand you a large amount of food. Just don't order that much, or split your meal with someone."

KEEP IT BASIC. "Walk down the street. That's what got me started. I didn't have to buy any expensive equipment. I didn't join any gyms."

MAKE YOUR JOB DO THE WORK. "I opened up a tree service. I can be outside and working and physical. And it helps to keep me in shape now."

BEAT FATIGUE. "If I'm tired or sluggish, a 10-minute walk or workout rejuvenates me, and I feel like I'm beginning a new day."

Part 4
Keeping That Belly Off

"Just Pill Me"

IT DOESN'T TAKE AN ADVANCED CHEMISTRY DEGREE TO FIGURE OUT that amphetamines help people lose weight. Drug addicts have known this for ages. So it would follow that ephedrine, an herbal stimulant with a chemical structure similar to that of amphetamines, would be a pretty effective weight-loss aid. (A note on terminology: The word *ephedra* is often used as a synonym for *ephedrine*, though the former is a plant source that contains the latter. In other words, ephedrine is derived from ephedra.)

If you've read anything about ephedrine recently, it was probably from one of two sources:

1. An ad for an ephedrine-and-caffeine supplement, showing pale, desperate-looking slobs transformed into bronzed, rippling Adonises and Adonisettes by the advertiser's magical pills.

2. A news article reporting that ephedrine causes heart attacks and strokes, and that the risks are utterly outrageous compared to the minuscule benefits.

If all you know about ephedrine products is what you've seen in those ads in bodybuilding magazines, you probably aren't aware that, in a 22-month period from 1997 to '99, the FDA received 140 complaints about adverse reactions to supplements containing ephedrine or similar compounds.

Belly Busters

▶▶ "People at work were shocked as they saw my transformation. My family was a little worried about my losing so much weight, but I assured them I wasn't doing anything illegal or unhealthy. That summer at the family reunion, some of my aunts and uncles didn't recognize me at first." ◀◀

—MARK OHLINGER
31, LOST 60 POUNDS

Conversely, if your only knowledge of ephedrine comes from your local newspaper, you most likely don't know that the stimulant has been strenuously researched at some of our most prestigious institutions, with the study results appearing in legitimate journals. We bet you've never heard that Frank Greenway, M.D., a prominent weight-loss researcher at the Pennington Biomedical Institute in Baton Rouge, Louisiana, wrote this in *Obesity Reviews* in 2001: "The peer-reviewed scientific literature suggests that the risks of caffeine and ephedrine are outweighed by the benefits of achieving and maintaining a healthy weight."

With the supplement industry portraying their wares as buffness-in-a-pill, and the news media labeling the products the weight-loss equivalent of Russian roulette, you can guess that the reality is somewhere in between.

Here's a closer look at the good and bad in fat-burning supplements.

THE DIT LIST

When you eat, you initiate a process called dietary-induced thermogenesis, or DIT, in which your body generates more energy, which produces heat, which burns calories. DIT accounts for about 10 percent of the calories you burn each day. Ephedrine-based products (which usually contain caffeine as well) are often described as *thermogenic* because they are also able to trigger this type of calorie burning.

The thermogenic effect, however, is only part of the reason why ephedrine-caffeine supplements work. About 75 percent of the benefit comes from appetite suppression, according to a 1993 study in the *International Journal of Obesity*. In plain and simple language, they help you eat less by mimicking your body's natural appetite suppressant, norepinephrine.

Over an extended period of time, that could lead to a whopping weight loss. To give just one example, a recent study of 180 obese people who took 20 milligrams of ephedrine and 200 milligrams of caffeine three times a day over a period of 6 months lost an average of 36 pounds.

As a bonus, the ephedrine-caffeine combo helps you preserve muscle while losing weight, so your body drops a higher percentage of fat than it would if you were simply dieting off the pounds. We can't overemphasize the importance of this. Say you start a diet at 260 pounds and lose 80 pounds, one-third of which is muscle. You have a sleeker silhouette but a slower metabolism than someone who has always been 180 pounds. If, instead, you had lost 80 pounds that consisted almost entirely of fat, you would actually have a faster metabolism than the average 180-pounder since more of your remaining body weight would be calorie-burning muscle.

A final benefit is that because ephedrine-caffeine supplements are stimulants, you could find that you have more productive workouts while using them. That would either increase your weight loss or add muscle to your frame while the supplements burn off your excess fat. Or both. (It's because such supplements are believed to improve performance that they have been banned by the Olympics, the NCAA, and other sports organizations.)

THERE MUST BE A CATCH

Indeed there is. There are several, in fact. First, ephedrine may prompt side effects including heart palpitations, slightly elevated blood pressure, dry mouth, and increased nervousness. That's because it switches on the same chemical mechanisms in your brain that trigger the fight-or-flight response your body experiences in dangerous situations. You get the same rush of anticipation you feel when you take money out of an ATM at midnight in a bad neighborhood.

Other potential problems are dizziness, insomnia, constipation, headaches, tremors, increased sweating, and depression.

Studies shows that the side effects tend to go away after 3 to 4 weeks of supplement use. Your body simply gets used to the stuff.

The jury is still out on the safety of ephedrine-caffeine supplements, at least according to the FDA and the National Institutes of Health's Office of Dietary Supplements. In particular, the Office of Dietary Supplements is currently working with the FDA and other federal government agencies to

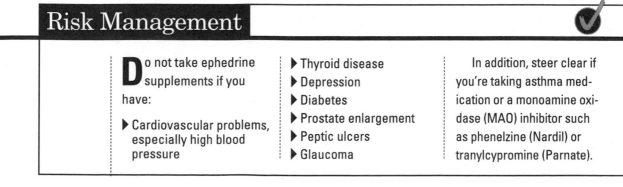

Risk Management

Do not take ephedrine supplements if you have:

▶ Cardiovascular problems, especially high blood pressure
▶ Thyroid disease
▶ Depression
▶ Diabetes
▶ Prostate enlargement
▶ Peptic ulcers
▶ Glaucoma

In addition, steer clear if you're taking asthma medication or a monoamine oxidase (MAO) inhibitor such as phenelzine (Nardil) or tranylcypromine (Parnate).

develop safety standards and guidelines for manufacturers of ephedrine-caffeine products.

The biggest problems occur when the wrong person takes ephedrine or when the right person takes too much. Side effects increase when the dosage reaches or exceeds 150 milligrams of ephedrine a day. The standard dosage is 60 milligrams a day, taken in three 20-milligram doses. Ninety milligrams is considered the safe upper limit.

As you can see in the "Risk Management" list on page 155, ephedrine is considered a big no-no for a lot of big-bellied men who may be overweight in part because of thyroid problems or depression (as discussed in

Muscle Builders for Fat Loss?

Since the Belly-Off diet includes whey protein, a traditional muscle-building supplement, should a guy trying to lose fat—especially abdominal fat—also consider taking creatine supplements?

Subjects in short-term creatine studies typically gain about 5 pounds; those in longer-term studies gain up to 9 pounds in 2 months. The weight gain is initially water that is pulled up into your muscles, making you feel like Superman the first couple weeks you use the supplement. After that, due to your ability to train harder and longer, you add Grade-A beef to your frame, with no more fat.

An open question is what would happen if you took creatine while decreasing the overall calories in your diet in an attempt to retain muscle while losing fat.

Researchers have looked at the issue several different ways. A 1998 study in the *European Journal of Applied Physiology* found that creatine helps retain muscle strength during a low-calorie diet. In 2001, a study in *Medicine and Science in Sports and Exercise* showed that creatine prevents the loss of muscle mass that normally occurs during weight loss. Another interesting finding in that study: The subjects using creatine while dieting were able to work harder in the weight room than the ones dieting without creatine.

If you put those two studies together and combine them with evidence showing that creatine prevents the muscle breakdown that occurs during normal exercise, you can reasonably conclude that supplementing would help you retain muscle size and strength as well as exercise intensity, even while you cut calories to lose weight. That means that after you'd dropped 10 or 20 or 30 pounds through diet, you'd still have the muscle size and strength

chapter 4). And if your abdominal fat has already made you diabetic, you're out of luck when it comes to thermogenics.

On the other hand, the supplements may even be recommended for some guys. If you feel cold most of the time, or at least after eating, you could have an impaired hormonal response to eating that prevents you from getting the normal DIT. A higher-protein diet will help, but a thermogenic supplement would help even more.

Our advice: Talk to your doctor before you take a thermogenic supplement. He may not know any more than what you've just read in this chapter (and he might not even know

you had before the weight loss. Plus, you'd be able to see your muscles better, since they'd be free of their veil of fat.

How to Get Loaded

Creatine works best with a "loading" phase in which you take in about 20 grams a day for 5 days, divided into four daily doses. After that, all you need for maintenance is 5 grams a day, following exercise. You don't even need to use it every day: Four or 5 days a week is probably fine.

To make sure you get all the benefits of the loading phase, you need to take each dose with 95 grams of pure sugar, or 75 grams of sugar and 25 grams of whey protein. That's 400 calories—most of it pure sugar—four times a day, for 5 days.

Despite all that sugar, there's a big difference between loading with creatine and loading with Twinkies. The point of the sugar is to deliberately spike your insulin to shuttle the creatine into your muscles, as opposed to inadvertently spiking insulin to indulge your sweet tooth. (*Note:* Don't load up on creatine if you have diabetes or a blood-sugar irregularity such as hypo- or hyperglycemia.)

You need to be careful about the other food you eat during the loading period: Take in about 1,000 calories a day through real food to go with the 1,600 calories of creatine, sugar, and whey protein.

If you decide to try creatine, you can get it in one of two ways: as a pure creatine monohydrate powder, or premixed with sugar (usually maltose or dextrose, not the sucrose in table sugar). After the loading phase, you don't have to worry about combining it with sugar. You can mix it in a post-workout shake with protein and whatever else you decide to put in there (fruit, frozen yogurt, milk).

Then watch your muscles grow, even as your belly shrinks.

this much). But he can at least rule out high blood pressure, thyroid disease, and an enlarged prostate. Also, ask whether he or someone he knows can recommend brands and companies that are trustworthy. A couple of products that have some good science behind them are Metabolife and Hydroxycut by MuscleTech, as well as Xenadrine.

TURN UP THE HEAT

If you decide to give an ephedrine-caffeine supplement a try, here's how to proceed.

▶ As suggested above, check with a doctor to make sure that these supplements are right for you and that you're free of health problems that would make the supplements dangerous. Get a resting EKG reading, and have a stress test done to make sure that you have no cardiovascular problems. (This is a good idea even if you aren't contemplating ephedrine supplements—especially if you're overweight and over 40.)

▶ The first time you buy a supplement, shop at GNC or a similar retailer. Ask the salesman for advice. Tell him you're looking for a product from the company that has the best reputation. Don't pretend you know any more than you do. If you're uncomfortable, if you don't think the salesman is giving you straight advice, or if you get the impression that his knowledge of thermogenics is more

limited than yours, leave and try someplace else.

▶ Look for a supplement that is standardized for 20 milligrams of ephedrine (derived from *ma huang*, which is the Chinese name for ephedra) or ephedra alkaloids, and 200 grams of caffeine (derived from guarana, an herbal caffeine source) per dose. Be aware that studies have shown the actual amount of ephedrine contained in supplements can vary significantly from what the label says. This can be a problem in two ways: You may not get enough of the active ingredients to derive the expected benefit, or you may get too much and unknowingly put yourself at greater risk of side effects.

▶ Follow the package directions to the letter. They should recommend three doses a day, and each dose should include several pills. A day's worth typically should be 9 to 12 pills. You'll probably be instructed to start with one dose a day for a week. If a dose is three pills, you'd take one pill three times a day. The second week, you'd take two pills three times a day; and the third week, you'd take the full load of three pills three times a day. Never exceed the recommended amounts. These are the doses that have been clinically tested to work well with minimal side effects. More is worse, not better.

▶ The directions will probably recommend taking the supplement 30 minutes before each meal. The only time to veer from these directions is if your final meal is within an hour or two of bedtime. Taking a dose with that meal would increase your risk of insomnia. Instead, take the supplement before a smaller meal 6 hours before bedtime, then have dinner at the usual time.

▶ For the first 3 to 4 weeks of treatment, you must take the supplement more than 1 hour before exercise. Ephedrine and caffeine may elevate your heart rate and blood pressure, which is also what exercise does. The two at once may not be a healthy combination.

▶ If you experience side effects that last more than 3 weeks, stop taking the supplement and check with a doctor.

▶ Don't combine ephedrine-and-caffeine supplements with any other stimulants, especially yohimbine. (Doing so could lead to a sharp increase in blood pressure.) You probably want to back off on your coffee or Diet Coke intake, too. Jitters have no upside. If you don't believe us, try asking your boss for a raise or an attractive woman for a date while shaking uncontrollably.

▶ Weigh the risks. Although, in our opinion, the dangers of ephedrine-caffeine supplements have been wildly overblown, the FDA has nonetheless received reports of some serious ephedrine-associated incidents, including strokes, heart attacks, and three deaths in a 22-month period between 1997 and 1999. When deciding whether to take an ephedrine-caffeine supplement, you have to ask yourself whether the risks and variables are more dangerous than your weight itself. If you have just a few pounds to lose, you may decide they aren't. (And you should know that no studies have been conducted on relatively lean men to see whether ephedrine-caffeine supplements work to get them extra-lean for beach season.)

▶ If you have a lot of weight to lose and no health risks, a supplement may be worth considering.

THE GREENING OF WEIGHT-LOSS SUPPLEMENTS

Two other weight-loss supplements showing some promise are fiber and green tea extract. Fiber acts by limiting your appetite, and a compound in green tea increases your metabolism and helps your body use more fat for energy. Here's a closer look at each.

Fiber. When you increase the fiber in your diet, you stay fuller between meals and even eat less at each meal. In addition, fiber helps control blood sugar and insulin.

The only side effects are gas and, perhaps, an extra visit to the bathroom each day. If you start slowly and gradually increase the fiber in your diet, you will easily be able to control any embarrassing incidents.

Foods such as fruits, vegetables, and whole grains are the best source of extra fiber, but if adding a lot of them to your diet means adding a lot of calories, you can go for fiber supplements, such as Metamucil. Take as directed on the package.

Green tea extract. A chemical in green tea called epigallocatechin gallate (its friends call it EGCG) can increase your total energy expenditure by 4 percent and promote fat burning. You could get the benefit from tea instead of EGCG supplements, but you'd have to drink 15 cups a day to get the effective dose of 90 milligrams, three times a day. And forget about getting this effect from black tea, which has one-tenth the EGCG of green.

As with fiber, green tea has multiple health benefits beyond fat loss. Its antioxidants are thought to help prevent cancer, and a 1993 Japanese study showed it could block the flu virus.

Once you get past those two, the evidence behind other fat-burning, appetite-curbing, fat-blocking supplements is pretty shaky. Here are three that have gotten some attention.

Chitosan. In theory, chitosan binds to fat in your intestine and prevents it from being absorbed. In one study, chitosan was compared to orlistat, the prescription fat-blocking drug discussed later in this chapter. The researchers examined fecal fat excretion (when they weren't updating their résumés, presumably) and found that orlistat indeed sends more fat down the poop chute, while chitosan doesn't. Another study found no weight loss with chitosan in 4 weeks of supplementation.

Of course, the whole idea that a fat blocker will prevent you from getting fat ignores a simple truth: Carbohydrates make you fat, too.

CLA. You have to like a supplement with a name that sounds like a super-secret government agency. And, like the CIA, conjugated linoleic acid goes in and out of favor. Some studies show no effect. For example, a 2000 study in the journal *Lipids* found that 3 grams a day of CLA for 2 months didn't affect anything—not muscle, fat, weight, metabolism, or the amount of fat versus carbohydrate used for energy.

A 2001 study in *International Journal of Obesity*, however, found that 4.2 grams a day produced a reduction in abdominal fat, with no reductions in overall body fat or lean tissue (muscle and everything else that isn't fat).

There's some smoke here—but no thermogenesis yet.

Pyruvate. Pyruvate is a weird one: It's a natural byproduct of exercise that somehow became a highly touted weight-loss supplement. While it seems to have some ability to reduce weight, the effective dose is extremely high: 22 grams a day, which is more than seven times the 3-gram dose recommended on product labels. Plus, you could end up with gas and diarrhea at such high doses. So you'd spend hundreds of dollars per month for a product that works in a mysterious way researchers can't identify.

PRESCRIPTION WEIGHT LOSS

When you consult with your doctor about whether weight-loss supplements are right for you, he may suggest prescription drugs such as sibutramine (Meridia) or orlistat (Xenical). You'd think that because they're prescription-only and doctor-recommended, they must work better than over-the-counter supplements. But the results of short- and long-term studies don't really show that.

Like ephedrine and caffeine, sibutramine works by putting the brakes on your appetite. A 1999 study in the *Journal of Obesity and Related Metabolic Disorders* found that subjects using sibutramine each lost a little more than 5 pounds in 8 weeks, versus a slight weight gain for a group taking a placebo.

Since you could easily get the same results with ephedrine-caffeine supplements, you'd think that sibutramine would at least cause fewer side effects. Again, that doesn't seem to be the case. In a recent long-term sibutramine study, 3 percent of the subjects had to drop out because of high blood pressure and increased heart rate.

In contrast, with long-term use, ephedrine and caffeine don't seem to increase blood pressure or heart rate—and might actually result in decreased blood pressure, according to studies published in the *International Journal of Obesity* in 1992 and 1994.

As for orlistat, it works by preventing your body from absorbing dietary fat. Instead of being digested and either stored in your gut or used for energy, fat moves straight on through. Gastrointestinal side effects are common, but on the bright side, they "decreas[e] considerably during the second year of treatment," according to a 2000 review in the journal *Heart Disease*.

And what do you get for your year of diarrhea, other than the promise of less diarrhea the second year? One long-term study showed weight loss of about 7½ pounds in trials lasting between 36 and 52 weeks. Compare that with the performance of the ephedrine-caffeine supplement Metabolife-356: It produced an average weight loss of 8.8 pounds in 8 weeks in a Columbia University study published in 2001 in the *International Journal of Obesity*.

Risley's Believe-It-or-Not

LIFE IN THE FAT LANE

Jesse Risley used to wonder how he could be an effective social studies teacher if he had a socially unacceptable physique.

His hobbies weren't entirely sedentary—he hunted and fished, and, living in the tornado belt, became a passionate storm chaser. But thanks to his equal passion for sodas, candy, pizza, fast food, ice cream, and Little Debbie snack cakes, this weather fanatic expanded like a weather balloon.

Risley began struggling with his weight when he was just 11. "I averaged out my weight gain over a 10-year period," he says. "Every year, I gained anywhere from 10 to 15 pounds."

Among the unpleasant consequences were headaches, body aches, fatigue, stomach upsets, and diarrhea, the last of which was brought on, he now believes, by eating too much greasy food. When he did get out and move, his stamina was nearly nonexistent and he was constantly short of breath.

When he got to college, he added another source of empty calories: beer. Just 2 years into his education, he had gone from big man on campus to really, really big man on campus. He wore size-42 pants and tipped the scales at 283 pounds.

"I felt bad about myself," he says. "People were afraid to make direct eye contact with me. Being that heavy, it was hard getting the girls."

THE TURNING POINT

For years, Jesse's doctor had advised him to lose weight. "Of course, the fat tooth in me just kind of ignored that," he says. "I thought I was young and invincible, and I could always lose the weight later."

Then, in May 2000, a physical exam showed that his triglycerides were off the charts. His cholesterol, blood pressure, and blood sugar were elevated, too.

"After eating sweets, I would crash; and in an hour, I would get very hungry and thirsty," he says. "Then I'd eat some more. It became a vicious cycle."

Finally, his doctor got tough. "He had a little talk with me," recalls Risley. "Since diabetes runs in my family, he told me that I needed to do something. I was on a crash course for major health problems."

It took one more nudge—a new photo on an ID card in March 2000—for him to accept that he had a problem. "Looking at that picture, I saw that I had a double chin and was just plain obese," he says. "It was a wake-up call."

Name: JESSE RISLEY
Date of Birth: August 1980
Residence: Streator, Illinois
Occupation: High school social studies teacher
Height: 6 foot 1

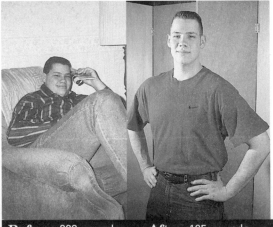

Before: 283 pounds   **After:** 195 pounds

THE PLAN OF ATTACK

Risley knew that his procrastinating days were over. He was looking at the immediate prospect of developing diabetes, heart disease, and perhaps dozens more obesity-related conditions—all before he even graduated from college.

Step one was research into nutrition. He quickly realized he was as addicted to junk food as alcoholics are to booze. So he went cold turkey, cutting out sugar, processed meats, and fast food. He began eating what he calls a natural-food diet high in protein, vegetables, and whole grains.

Instead of snacking on a Snickers bar, he would grab a hard-boiled egg, a handful of peanuts, or a piece of fruit. "The first week or so, I had terrible cravings. But soon I felt better than I had in years," he says.

Water played a big role in his plan. Each day, he topped off his tank with as much as 100 ounces—about 3 quarts. He also took to the streets, walking 3 to 5 miles a day, 5 to 7 days a week.

He lost 50 pounds by October 2000.

"When you're obese, you lose weight more rapidly at first," he says. "Since then, It's come off a little more slowly." Not until summer 2001 did he reach his current weight: 195 pounds.

Still, he wasn't completely satisfied with his appearance. Although he was no longer a fat guy, he was still flabby. So he joined a gym and teamed with a personal trainer who set up a strength-training program for him. He now lifts weights 3 or 4 nights a week, rotating upper- and lower-body workouts and concentrating on his midsection. He also started a regimen of high-intensity interval training.

"I'm starting to tone up a little bit," he says. "But I'd still like to take off another 5 or 10 pounds."

LIFE IN THE FIT LANE

Now that he has shed nearly 100 pounds, Risley's aches, pains, stomach upsets, and fatigue are gone. His blood chemistry and blood pressure are normal.

Hunting is easier, with his added strength and endurance. "I'm able to go with just a little bit more spunk in me," he says.

Weight loss also helped him in another type of hunt: His female classmates at Illinois State University liked what they saw. "It's helped my social life quite a bit," he says. "I've had a couple of girlfriends, and I've gotten compliments from a lot of people."

Other people asked if he was ill. He deflected such comments with a classic understatement: "I'm feeling all right."

His next step is one he never contemplated as an out-of-shape teenager: He plans to become an assistant coach for one of the high school sports teams.

HIS TIPS

BEWARE OF YOUR "FAT" TOOTH. "I'm a firm believer that it exists, because I've had it."

EDUCATE YOURSELF. "Before I learned more about food, I just thought, 'If it's on the market, it must be safe. They'd tell us if it was bad for us.' In fact, some of it is bad for us. It's a big reason why more and more people, especially young people, are gaining weight."

GET OFF YOUR BUTT NOW. "If you don't take care of your body when you're young, you're going to be sorry when you're older. I've talked to a lot of older guys who wish they had gotten in shape 20 or 30 years ago so they wouldn't be beating themselves to death now to lose 50 or 60 pounds."

CHAPTER 15

Desperate Measures

Each year, thousands—if not millions—of Americans fall for the notion that they can buy a shortcut to slimness. They spend money on ab rollers, electronic muscle stimulators, liposuction, even stomach stapling.

None of these strategies works the way you think it will. Oh, you'll definitely end up a little lighter—in the wallet. But you might also end up paying for a shortcut with your life.

MISSING THE SPOT

Perhaps the most widespread and enduring myth in the entire fitness industry is the idea that exercising a specific area of your body will cause fat to disappear from that area. It makes intuitive sense. For example, when you want to trim some shrubs in your front yard, you don't start the job by cutting down a tree out back. You grab the hedge clippers and head straight out to those azaleas. Likewise, when you want to trim your gut, you don't automatically think, "I'll eat less food while steadily increasing my volume of exercise and building muscle to speed up my metabolism." Your instinct is to go directly to the site of the problem. Hence, the commercial success of ab rollers.

Working your abdominal muscles is not entirely a waste of energy—there are some perfectly fine reasons to build a firm, strong midsection. But the 5 minutes you spend doing that won't have anywhere near the gut-busting impact that you could get with an hour of running or weight lifting.

Consider this: University of Virginia researchers calculated that it would take 250,000 crunches to burn 1 pound of fat—that's 100 crunches a day for 7 years.

And you don't get any say as to where that pound of fat comes from. It could very well come from your gut—visceral abdominal fat is far more likely than subcutaneous fat to be burned by exercise. Then again, it might not. Where you gain fat and where you lose it is determined by genetics, not by which muscles you exercise.

Here's an example that brings home the point: If spot reduction were anatomically possible, tennis players' racket arms would contain less fat than their inactive arms. Yet a study of 20 players who hit the courts for at least 6 hours a week showed that both arms contained about the same amount of fat. The racket arms were significantly more muscular—as you'd expect—but no leaner.

Abdominal exercises have their place in a workout program. But if you're serious about losing your gut, ab moves should never be the main attraction.

SHOCKINGLY USELESS

We can have a bit of respect for a guy who thinks 5 minutes of ab rolling will give him a smaller midsection. At least he's acknowledging the importance of those 5 minutes. But a guy who believes that electrical muscle stimulation (EMS) will produce meaningful changes in his body is in a different category. He wants the appearance of having done hard work without actually doing any.

Here's the theory behind EMS: You put electrodes on your muscles to induce involuntary twitches, and allegedly you'll walk away with bigger muscles and a smaller waist. In reality, the machines don't work as advertised. A 2001 study at the University of Wisconsin–La Crosse put 27 college students on either EMS or a machine that delivered no current. After 8 weeks, the EMS group showed no differences in strength, weight, or waist size. (Curiously, the group getting no electrical stimulation actually got a bit stronger and lost a small amount of weight.)

Another problem with EMS is that it reinforces the perception that technology can solve every problem that

Belly Busters

▶▶ "Although it has not been easy, I have learned one thing: There are no miracle cures for weight loss. It only takes a proper diet and exercise." ◀◀

—JOE REPOSA
38, LOST 52 POUNDS

man creates for himself. So you ate too much, exercised too little, and ended up with a 42-inch waist. No problem—here's a machine that will shock away the fat and replace it with muscle.

There is some science behind EMS. It's been used in physical rehabilitation for years, with genuine results. For example, EMS has been shown to help patients regain strength in their leg muscles following major knee surgery. So it works for particular muscle groups immobilized by traumatic injury. If your muscles are healthy and fully ambulatory, however, EMS will prove about as stimulating as 3 hours of C-SPAN. Also keep in mind that rehabilitative effects are created by large consoles designed for clinical use, not the little boxes offered in infomercials.

LEAVE THE FAT, TAKE THE CANNULA

The concept of attacking fat reservoirs via a surgical strike holds a lot of appeal—at least for the more than 50,000 American men who had liposuction in 2000. (And for each of those guys, 6 women had the surgery.)

The technique itself would make for a pretty good scene in a horror movie. Usually, the doctor uses a tumescent-fluid method, in which he injects large volumes of fluid into the fat deposits targeted for removal. The fluid consists of salt water, epinephrine (also known as adrenaline, a hormone that constricts blood vessels and minimizes bleeding), and lidocaine (an anesthetic that dulls pain enough for some patients to forgo general anesthesia).

The doctor then makes a tiny incision in the skin and inserts a hollow suction tube called a cannula to manually loosen and suck away the fat. Since the fat inevitably contains some blood, it has the consistency and color of a strawberry milkshake.

Some practitioners remove up to 20 pounds of fat at a time. As you can imagine, the more fat a doctor removes, the higher the risk involved. That's why the usual recommendation is to perform liposuction in a hospital anytime more than 11 pounds is scheduled for removal.

For smaller sucks, the surgery can be performed in a doctor's office or an outpatient medical center. But that brings up another point: Although plastic surgeons perform most liposuctions, the procedure can legally be performed by any M.D. (You should be particularly suspicious if your ophthalmologist pulls out a cannula.)

Liposuction is major surgery that carries major risks, including death. Since liposuction "incidents" aren't reportable, however, it's impossible to know how many people are injured or killed as a result of the procedure. One doctor-owned malpractice carrier conducted an unscientific survey of plastic surgeons and found that 69 liposuction-related deaths were reported in an 18-month period in 1997 and '98. Some experts say that figure is too low, while others believe it's too high. Some estimate that for every death there are 15 to 20 serious injuries.

Of all the ways to die, surely death by unnecessary cosmetic procedure must rank as one of the most embarrassing. Consider the 51-year-old Florida man who died after an almost 10-hour surgery that included liposuction and penile enlargement.

Though the vast majority of liposuctions produce happier outcomes, a lot can go wrong. Fatal complications can include:

▶ Cardiac arrest

▶ Toxic drug reactions including respiratory arrest, cardiac arrhythmias, and convulsions (our 51-year old Floridian friend reportedly died from an overdose of anesthetic, although the medical examiner initially determined he succumbed to heart damage caused by taking diet drugs prior to surgery)

▶ Fluid overload, which can cause congestive heart failure and pulmonary edema (fluid buildup in the lungs)

▶ Hypotension (abnormally low blood pressure caused by shock)

▶ Deep-vein thrombosis (blood clots that reach the lungs)

▶ Necrotizing fasciitis (a painful infection caused by flesh-eating bacteria that spread beneath the skin)

Even if you survive, you still risk the following nonfatal complications.

▶ Ischemic optic neuropathy (blindness in one or both eyes caused by anemia or hypotension)

▶ Bacterial infections of the skin and soft tissue

▶ Accidental perforation of intestines (you could be at especially high risk if you have an undiagnosed hernia)

If these aren't good enough reasons to keep your distance from a cannula, consider this: Liposuction *does not* reduce your risk of heart disease or other conditions associated with excess belly fat. There's no evidence that it produces any beneficial metabolic changes.

That's because it removes only the relatively benign subcutaneous fat in your love handles and on top of your abdominal muscles. The most dangerous fat, the visceral goo surrounding your internal organs, remains untouched. (The same is true of apronectomy, a surgical procedure that removes an "apron" of belly fat.)

That leaves only one benefit of liposuction: You look better in the area that was liposucked. Unfortunately, there's no guarantee you'll look good forever. Writes British clinical medicine professor Peter Kopelman, M.D., in the *International Journal of Obesity,* "In most circumstances, [cosmetic fat-removing procedures] are followed by rapid replacement of the extracted adipose tissue with weight regain." You won't regain the weight in the same places, since the fat cells have been permanently removed from those spots. But it may show up someplace where you'll like it even less.

Plastic surgeons say the ideal lipo patient is someone who is already in good shape and wants to take out some stubborn pockets of fat that remain after years of healthful eating and exercise. In fact, one procedure that's increasingly popular with men is ab-etching, in which fat cells are removed in a way that brings out the abdominal six-pack. However, you need to go into the surgery with well-developed muscles beneath the fat. Otherwise, there isn't much point.

Death of a Drug Dealer

One of history's most notorious plastic-surgery disasters took place on July 4, 1997. The scene was a Mexico City hospital. The patient was Amado Carrillo Fuentes, then the world's most powerful drug lord.

Carrillo had good reasons for wanting to alter his appearance. During the late 1980s and early 1990s, he allegedly moved tons of cocaine from South America to Mexico in Boeing 727s and cargo aircraft, then shipped it by truck across the U.S. border. He and his organization reportedly grossed an estimated $4 million to $5 million a day, and by the mid-'90s Carrillo was a billionaire.

In what is believed to have been a desperate attempt to change his identity, Carrillo underwent 8 hours of cosmetic surgery on his face and liposuction on his midsection.

The operation didn't go as planned. Carrillo died in his hospital room, possibly from a postoperative heart attack, although Mexican authorities refused to rule out foul play. His bruised corpse was flown to his childhood home in northern Mexico and laid out in a silk-lined coffin. Among the mourners were hundreds of reported drug-world associates.

They were not in a friendly mood.

In November 1997, according to the *Washington Post*, police found three 66-gallon oil drums near a highway, each containing a bound-and-gagged body embedded in concrete. The victims were identified as the doctors who had operated on Carrillo. Just 5 days before, Mexico's federal drug agency had issued arrest warrants for the doctors on the suspicion that they had intentionally killed Carrillo.

The discovery of the doctors' bodies allowed authorities to declare the case closed.

So ended one of history's most unusual malpractice episodes.

A TIE THAT BINDS YOUR APPETITE

If you're more than 100 pounds overweight, you may have considered gastric-bypass surgery, sometimes called stomach stapling. An estimated 40,000 Americans have gotten clamped, most of them women (including singer Carnie Wilson, whose 1999 surgery can be viewed on the Internet via streaming video).

Surgeons have developed dozens of gastric-bypass procedures. The one most commonly performed in the United States is the Roux-en-Y, named after the French surgeon who developed it. In this procedure, a segment of small intestine is attached to a small pouch created at the top of your stomach. This causes food to bypass most of your stomach and the first part of your small intestine.

The change in your life is instant and dramatic. With one procedure, your stomach goes from a tank that can hold 2 to 3 pounds of food to a Dixie cup capable of holding just 1 to 2 ounces. That's about five bites. It's impossible to eat as much as you did before, and much of the food you do eat isn't absorbed.

Not surprisingly, most people who have the surgery end up losing an enormous amount of weight. The Swedish Obese Subjects study, which has tracked 1,600 patients since 1992, shows that gastric-bypass recipients are considerably thinner than obese patients who enrolled in conventional diet-and-exercise programs.

Specific benefits of the surgery include an average weight loss of 66 pounds, a 60 percent decrease in insulin levels, a 25 percent decrease in glucose and triglycerides, and a 10 percent reduction in blood pressure. Researchers also calculated that patients have a 14-fold reduced risk of developing diabetes.

But gastric-bypass surgery is hardly a free lunch. Even proponents of the procedure say the risks and side effects are so serious that it should be considered only as a last resort.

Patients pay a heavy price, especially at first. Risks of the surgery itself include internal hemorrhaging, massive infection, and a lengthy recuperation. And then there are the lifestyle changes. Among them:

Microscopic meals. Instead of sitting down to three squares a day, you have to graze on bite-size portions that you must chew until they're practically liquefied.

"Dumping." If you eat just one bite too many—or any sweets at all—you can experience a syndrome that includes sweating, nausea, diarrhea, faintness, and dizziness.

Nutritional deficiencies. You're likely to absorb less calcium and fewer B vitamins and other essential nutrients. Some experts also worry about long-term gastrointestinal effects.

Depression. The Swedish Obese Subjects study found that gastric-bypass patients were in better physical and mental condition than the people who were pursuing weight loss the old-fashioned way. But some staplees end

Belly Busters

▶▶ "Excuses like 'I have no time; I'm too tired, too old, too weak' are just that . . . excuses. Nothing just happens without effort. It is because of constant effort and education that this occurred, and I am glad I found the strength to do it." ◀◀

—RAFFAEL BORELLI
34, LOST 40 POUNDS

up clinically depressed. In theory, it seems simple to give up holiday meals with your family, candlelit dinners with your spouse, and beer-fueled tailgate parties with your buddies. But in reality, some guys end up mourning these lost chances to bond over food and drink.

We know, we know . . . you're worried that even if you keep your digestive system intact, a diet and workout schedule will force you to give up eating, drinking, and being merry. That's not the case, we promise. The next chapter will tell you how you can get a flatter belly while having your cake and eating it, too.

Belly Off SUCCESS STORY

A Rock-'n'-Roll Revelation

LIFE IN THE FAT LANE

Dennis Vaughn looks at his 4-year-old son and sees the spitting image of himself as a boy: a skinny kid with energy to spare. This makes him wonder how he wound up so much like his own dad, a heavyset type-2 diabetic. "People would say, 'You look just like your father'—and they weren't referring to our faces," says Vaughn.

It wasn't all that tough to figure out how it happened. Four years of college plus 2 more in grad school took their toll. "Too much partying, too much studying," says Vaughn. "There wasn't time to do anything else." Then came work, marriage, and a family.

By the time he was 32, Vaughn had morphed from lanky kid to lardy guy—265 pounds to be exact, wearing size-44 pants. He suffered from mysterious headaches. To top it off, his doctor diagnosed him with high blood pressure and a fairly high cholesterol level of 225.

THE TURNING POINT

Vaughn realized he was headed for trouble when he considered that obesity and diabetes type 2 run in his family, affecting both his father and his maternal grandmother. "My grandmother had part of a leg amputated. That scared me," he says.

The final turning point came one August night in 2000. "I'm embarrassed to admit it, but it was at a Mötley Crüe concert," he says. He went to every concession stand in the arena, looking to buy a tour T-shirt—but couldn't find one that was big enough to fit him.

"That was the last straw," says Vaughn. "I was too fat."

THE PLAN OF ATTACK

The very next day, Vaughn started a carb-restricted diet. Having been repeatedly disappointed by low-fat schemes that never worked, he says, "I *(continued)*

Name: DENNIS VAUGHN
Occupation: Crisis services supervisor for a community mental-health program
Residence: Luray, Virginia
Date of Birth: October 1967
Height: 5 foot 10

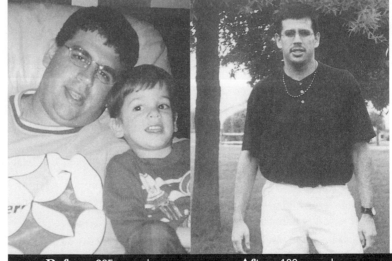

Before: 265 pounds   **After:** 169 pounds

decided a diet that allowed me to eat meat and cheese couldn't be all bad."

During the first 2 weeks, Vaughn suffered major cravings for all the stuff he'd been denying himself: chips, doughnuts, bread, sugar, and the like. However, he lost 16 pounds, which outweighed the cravings. "It was nice to see something immediate," he says. "It was definitely motivating."

Soon after he blacklisted carbs, Vaughn checked with his physician, who suggested he wait until he'd lost more weight before starting heavy-duty exercise. "I did a little bit of walking, but nothing I would consider a formal exercise program," he says.

Finally, after 4 months, he had dropped a total of 40 pounds. Only then did he feel ready to tackle fitness.

"That December, I got a subscription to *Men's Health*. Included with my first issue was an exercise poster that focused on arms, abs, and chest exercises." Vaughn set up a couple of dumbbells and a mat in his bedroom, and adapted the poster so that he could alternate upper-body, abs, and leg workouts during the week. On the days in between, he tossed in a little Tae Bo, some mountain biking, or running.

In just over a year, Vaughn cut nearly 100 pounds from his frame, shaving almost 12 inches from his waist.

LIFE IN THE FIT LANE

Almost immediately after Vaughn changed to a low-carbohydrate diet, his cholesterol plunged to 175. Unfortunately, he still has high blood pressure. "My doctor now feels it's hereditary," he says.

Vaughn believes his health has benefited in other ways, too. His headaches are a thing of the past, he doesn't get sick as often, and he feels more energetic. "My goal at some point is to run a 10-K, just to say I've done it. I think I can do it now," he says.

The oddest part about losing all the weight? "There was actually a rumor spreading a couple of months ago that I was terminally ill, which I kind of took personally because I think I look pretty darn good and healthy," says Vaughn.

And at least now no one can accuse him of being Mötley Crüe's biggest fan.

HIS TIPS

STAY HOME. "I made a conscious decision not to join a gym, because I know me and it would be easy not to do it. The gym is across town, and if I don't go, I can forget about it. But I go to my bedroom every night. It's kind of hard to get away from it."

KEEP RECORDS. "I kept a log from the first day . . . how many reps, how many sets. And if I miss a day, I write that in there, too, and why. I usually do my workout in the morning before work, and if I'm running late, [my log is] a good reminder when I go home. It bothers me to leave [the log] empty, so I'll go and finish in the evening. So I don't have anything hanging over my head."

DON'T WORRY ABOUT WHAT OTHER PEOPLE THINK. "My mother takes a little offense that I don't eat everything on the table. It just takes time for people to get adjusted to the changes. They have to learn it's not an insult to them. It's not that you don't like their cooking. It's putting health first."

You
versus
the World

MOST GUYS STRUGGLE WITH THE DESIRE FOR A PERFECT LIFE. Each of us wants the perfect job, the perfect marriage, the perfect body honed by the perfect diet and the perfect exercise program.

The problem is that, even if perfection were attainable in even one of these areas, it would preclude achieving it in any of the others. The perfect job would be so complex that you wouldn't have time or energy for a perfect marriage. Likewise, you could never create the perfect marriage and still have energy for even a good job, much less a perfect one.

And in almost any career or marital scenario, there'd be little time left over for building that perfect body. A life built around counting calories, working out, and playing your favorite sports would compromise your work and marriage, each of which would already be compromised by the presence of the other. (Hell, we bet just watching your favorite sports sometimes gets you into trouble with the wife.) And forget about adding "perfect" kids to the mix.

So chances are, not one aspect of your life will ever turn out perfectly. There are probably parts of your life you don't like. You most likely struggle at being a husband and father. You may occasionally screw up workouts and accomplish less than you know you could. Once in a while, you'll eat enough sugar to put a horse into a diabetic coma. On your worst days, you might do lousy work, argue with your wife, mess up your workout, then go home to eat ice cream and yell at your kids.

But there's one useful lesson that comes of falling short of the standards you set for yourself: You can always do better the next day. Poor work can be revised, or at least not repeated. Spouses and children can be apologized to and treated better. A bad workout can often be a sign that it's time to shift some things around, to try something new or go back to something that worked in the past. And your body really does forgive you for a few poor food choices. With enough water and a day's worth of good food, you can usually undo the damage.

One bad day, in other words, doesn't undo a good program. Remember this to avoid having 2 bad days in a row. And if you have 2, fight like hell to avoid having a third.

Belly Busters

▶▶ "I feel fantastic about how I look and feel. I feel a renewed sense of confidence and well-being. I feel that there is nothing I cannot overcome or accomplish." ◀◀

—DARYN HOBAL
31, LOST 30 POUNDS

Here are some of the scenarios in which it will be hardest for you to stick to your diet-and-exercise program. Hopefully, this will help you see the problem coming and avoid having a bad day in the first place. At the very least, we hope to help you prevent a single off day from becoming 2 or 3.

YOU VERSUS YOUR SCHEDULE

A lot of guys are convinced that they're so busy they can't possibly find time to exercise. Usually, that just means they haven't really looked. Here are some ideas to help you find a little time you didn't know you had. Even if you have plenty, there's no need to waste any of it. Use these suggestions to make your workouts more time-efficient.

Don't waste transit time. Before you join a gym, locate it on a map. Also pinpoint your home and workplace. If the routes between the three destinations form a triangle, don't buy that membership—you'll find it hard to go out of your way to the gym. Look for a health club that's a straight shot from home and work, or at least find one that's very close by.

Don't waste warmup time. Perhaps the most worthless piece of workout advice is the old "Warm up for 5 to 10 minutes on a stationary bike or treadmill." Unless you're going to ride or run for your entire workout, such a start-up is a near-complete waste of time. The point of a warmup is to increase your core temperature. But core temperature rises gradually for the first 30 minutes of exercise—you can't just crank it up with a quick jog on a treadmill.

Your muscles, on the other hand, really can warm up in 5 to 10 minutes. So it makes a lot more sense to focus on them in your warmup. You can do this one of two ways. If you're doing circuit routines such as the ones in chapter 11, one warmup circuit will work just fine. Pick weights you think you can use for 20 repetitions, and do 10 to 12 reps of each exercise at a slow, steady pace. You warm up your muscles and connective tissues, and you get your neurological system prepared for the lifts as well.

Or use this method in your workouts: Start with a light stretch (as we said in chapter 13, you can ignore the "Never stretch a cold muscle" advice if you don't stretch aggressively past the point of discomfort). Then do abdominal exercises, followed by 3 to 4 warmup sets of the first exercise in your routine.

Don't waste workout time. A lot of guys walk into gyms fancying themselves instant bodybuilders. They find routines in hardcore bodybuilding magazines that call for multiple sets of three or four exercises for each muscle group. So a novice lifter will be doing 10 sets for his biceps and another 10 for his triceps.

Many studies have found that beginners make about as much progress doing one set of each exercise as they do with multiple sets. You do need to perform more sets as you get more advanced, to keep building strength and muscle size. But you'll probably never hit a point

Belly Busters

▶▶"When I see people I haven't seen in a few years, they say, 'Oh my God. How'd you do it?' And it just feels so good."◀◀

—STEVEN KLAPOW
32, LOST 57 POUNDS

where double-digit sets for any particular muscle group isn't overkill.

And even when you've progressed to multiple sets, you're far better off reserving the big number for the big muscles. That means doing squats and deadlifts instead of leg presses and leg curls; shoulder presses instead of lateral raises; and bench presses instead of chest flies. When practical, choose exercises that work more than one joint—your elbows and shoulders instead of just your shoulders, for example.

Don't waste your body's best moments. Most guys have to exercise before or after work. Exercise before work and you have a sense of accomplishment before you start your official workday. Exercise after work and you'll probably find you can perform better since your body temperature will be a little higher before your workout begins. But the performance issue is secondary to adherence. Choose the time that works best for you, so you'll stick with it and benefit from it.

Don't lose track of your stuff. On average, men spend about 6 weeks a year just looking for stuff. So make sure your exercise gear is always at hand by packing your gym bag the night before each workout. Set it by the door or stash it in your car, so you can't forget it. You might even keep a spare bag of gear in the trunk or at work, in case you do forget.

You can make a better go of your diet, too, if you reorganize your fridge and kitchen cabinets. One trick: Keep your fresh vegetables on the top shelf of the refrigerator, as close to eye-level as you can get them. Put the beer and snack stuff in the vegetable crisper. Trust us, you won't forget where you put them. Stowing the vegetables guarantees they'll rot before you remember to eat them.

YOU VERSUS BAD WEATHER

Leave it to a good blizzard to bring your exercise program to a grinding halt. A heat wave can also do the trick. A day or two without exercise isn't the end of the world, especially when the weather poses a bigger threat to your health than a lack of exercise. When a day or two stretches into a week or two, you start to lose the benefits you worked so hard to accrue.

Miss a few workouts and you'll start to get a little cranky. Go a week without exercise and you'll have trouble con-

centrating at work and sleeping at night. After 2 weeks without exercise, your aerobic-fitness level will have declined by 4 to 6 percent. Research shows that strength performance stays with you a little longer than aerobic fitness, so you'll retain most of your strength for up to 4 weeks of inactivity. Your muscular endurance, however, will probably decline quite a bit, so you'll be able to lift as much but you won't be able to do as many sets and repetitions. If you give up working out altogether, your fitness levels will return to your pre-exercise baseline within 2 to 8 months—the higher your level, the longer it'll take for it to waste away entirely.

These tips should help you keep moving, no matter what obstacles the weatherman throws your way.

Welcome Jack Frost. Think of that nip in the air as an exercise tool rather than a roadblock. You can actually get a more effective aerobic workout in the winter than in the summer, since you won't dehydrate and overheat as quickly. Some research suggests that cold weather causes your body to work harder since your heart has to pump blood faster to keep you warm and moving.

The key to exercising in cold weather is layering your clothes. Wear enough gear that you feel warm but not too hot and sweaty. If you perspire too much, you'll become drenched and at risk for hypothermia. In fact, you lose heat 26 times faster when you're wet. So invest in a good water-resistant, breathable shell jacket, and you may actually enjoy exercising in the winter.

 Belly Busters

▶▶ "Even though I am 58, I feel as good as I did in my 30s." ◀◀

—BILL STEPHENSON
LOST 43 POUNDS

Beware his cousin, Eddie Asthma. Two recent European studies suggest that exercising in cold weather may lead to lung damage. In particular, endurance athletes who train in harsh winter environments have three times the risk of asthma and a 25 percent greater chance of developing bronchitis. You can avoid these problems by warming up indoors first (try some jumping jacks and stretches) and wearing a scarf or mask to warm the air before it enters your lungs.

If life gives you snow, make a snowman. The most strenuous outdoor workouts you can get come during snow season. Snow shoveling tests the endurance of your back muscles, and dragging your kids around the yard on a sled kicks your ass. Some guys like to go even further and do official exercise. The benefits are amazing: A 170-pound guy can burn about 615 calories in an hour of cross-country skiing and 540 calories in an hour of downhill skiing. Snowshoeing burns even more: about 735 calories an hour.

Go easy on the comfort food. Studies have shown that appetite really does increase during the coldest months, for both psychological and physiological reasons. Food makes us feel more secure and protected from the bad weather outside. So stock up on hearty soups. The warmth of the soup has an obvious psychological benefit, and research has shown that foods with a high liquid content make you feel full sooner than more solid foods.

Limit heat exposure. Summer has its pitfalls, too. The death of an NFL player and several college athletes in the summer of 2001 should serve as a wake-up call. If highly trained athletes can collapse and die from heat-related illness, what about the rest of us?

Your first line of defense against heatstroke is time. The first few times you exercise outdoors in high heat or humidity, keep the workouts short—only 15 to 20 minutes. Add time as you become acclimated. You'll know you're acclimated when you finish a mid-July workout without spending the rest of the day feeling as if you'd been pulled through a wringer. Add a few minutes per workout, and back off if you feel wrung out again.

When possible, avoid exercising outdoors between 10:00 A.M. and 3:00 P.M. We say "when possible" because a guy who likes to run at noon (like president George W. Bush) is going to do it no matter what the weather is like.

Finally, seek shade during outdoor workouts, or at least stay off tracks or streets with tarred surfaces. Wooded areas are always a good bet.

On bad-air days, take it inside. A recent European study suggests it may be a bad idea to exercise outdoors on certain days in the summer. "Code orange" weather occurs when summer heat mixes with air pollution. This nasty brew can damage even a healthy, active guy's lungs.

When faced with code-orange days (you should be able to find smog reports in the local media), find another

Belly Busters

▶▶▶ "This is a lifestyle change. All things are okay in moderation. I avoid fatty foods, but now and then can afford to treat myself because I keep up my end of the bargain—and exercise." ◀◀

—MARK OHLINGER
31, LOST 60 POUNDS

exercise venue. If you don't have access to a gym, work out in the early morning or evening, and avoid heavily trafficked areas. Sunday mornings are often less smoggy than weekdays or Saturday mornings.

YOU VERSUS SOCIAL SITUATIONS

It's normal to want to celebrate special occasions with food and drink. The problem is, damned near every day is a special occasion for somebody, and we end up with access to celebratory food and drink far more often than we need or want to.

There is a middle ground between bacchanalian indulgence and monkish abstinence. It's not a big middle ground, but it's there.

Master strategic starters. Have a healthy, appetite-quenching appetizer. One study found that women who had a soup appetizer consumed about 100 fewer total calories at lunch, and they didn't eat more at dinner or feel hungrier later.

Another good starter is low-fat or fat-free tortilla chips with spicy guacamole and salsa. The chips are worthless calories, so eat just a few and pile

the guacamole on thick: The avocadoes in it are rich in monounsaturated fat that helps improve blood-lipid profiles, reduce your risk of heart disease, and make you feel fuller longer.

Limit yourself to one drink per day. By now, everyone must know about the research showing a drink or two a day prevents heart disease in men. More than that raises your risk of high blood pressure, stroke, heart failure, and a number of other undesirable conditions. You should also remember that alcohol has calories. If you take in 150 calories in the form of a beer, try to cut 150 calories somewhere else. Here are five foods that are roughly 150 calories.

▶ 30 cheese crackers

▶ 1 ounce of peanuts

▶ 1 ounce of cashews

▶ 7½ ounces of tortilla chips

▶ 2 nachos supreme

Don't drink and operate culinary machinery. A study at Laval University in Quebec City found that the calories in alcohol do nothing to satisfy your appetite. Your body's hunger mechanism is blind to alcohol. So you take in 150 calories per beer, 106 calories per 5-ounce glass of red wine, or roughly 587 calories per White Russian—and you don't feel any fuller than before you had a drink.

Plus, the calories you get from food while you're drinking are even more likely to be stored as fat because your body metabolizes alcohol preferentially, meaning it ignores the food as it tries to rid itself of the booze. And where do you think it stores that alcohol-induced fat? Oh, yeah, we covered that way back in chapter 4. You knew there was a good story behind the phrase *beer belly*.

YOU VERSUS THE HOLIDAYS

Holidays aren't as tough on your waist as you've been led to believe. A recent study by the National Institutes of Health tracked 200 men and women from late September to early March. On average, people who weren't trying to lose weight gained only 0.8 pound during the holidays, although many believed they'd gained four times as much. The subjects who reported more physical activity during the holidays actually lost 1.5 pounds, while the less active ones gained 1.5 pounds.

The following strategies should help you get through eggnog season with your waistline intact.

Don't skip meals. Even if you sleep in your own bed throughout the holidays, you probably do all your normal activities—wake up, eat, go to bed—at different times. It's easy to skip your normal bowl of Wheaties when you wake up at 10:00 instead of 7:00, and few of us are going to stop and eat lunch at noon when we know the holiday feast commences at 3:00. But we still eat—those Christmas cookies sure hit the spot, and the eggnog washes them down just fine.

You have to see this problem coming and, whenever possible, grab a normal meal. Even if it's just soup or a slice of peanut-butter toast, you'll shut down your hunger and eat fewer calories for a while—which may be enough to get you past the cookie tray.

Feast responsibly. There are few things in life more pleasurable than sitting around a table with your family and making a lot of food disappear. Still, you can prioritize the food by degree of pleasure. The meat is the main attraction, so if you start with a lot of it, you'll automatically eat less of everything else. Add some vegetables and a little gravy and stuffing, and you're probably full—meaning you can skip the roll and butter, mashed potatoes, and Jell-O mold.

Dessert? Don't deprive yourself by taking the sliver of pie meant for Grandma while your brother eats a slice the size of his shoe. You'll feel self-conscious, you'll resent your diet, and you'll just sneak into the kitchen in the middle of the night and eat the leftover pie anyway. So eat what looks good to you, and get it over with. However, if you have a lot of dessert choices, you may find that a little of everything works better than a lot of a couple things. You'll enjoy them more and take in less total food.

Remember that water is your friend, especially if there's a lot of alcohol at the table. Drink as much H_2O as you can.

Get off the couch. If you're like most guys, the recliner starts calling your name 5 minutes after the last forkful of pecan pie. This is an evolutionary mechanism designed to keep us from being dragooned into dish duty. But here's a better idea: Herd the family out to the backyard for touch football. Or tell Mom and Dad that you love being back in the old neighborhood and have your heart set on walking over to 85th Street to see what the new folks did to the O'Malley place. Whatever the excuse, a half-hour walk will make you feel a lot better than would a 2-hour nap.

YOU VERSUS BUSINESS TRAVEL

A lot of guys simply give up when they're on the road. You can't pull out a measuring cup in a restaurant and figure exactly how much they've put on your plate. You can't walk into a gym in Tacoma and expect to find the exact same equipment you have in your gym back home in Pacoima.

And if it's a short trip with little downtime, it may do more harm than good to watch every bite you eat and squeeze in a workout when you're physically and mentally exhausted from travel. Stress, as we saw in chapter 4, can do as much damage to your waistline as bad food or a missed workout. It may make more sense to take a long shower, eat some comfort food, and catch up on your sleep.

On the other hand, healthful food and exercise can take some of the edge off that stress. So let's look at some of the ways you can travel light.

Pack right. Before you leave, you can't anticipate all the exercise options that'll be available to you. You may want to let your mood decide which option you'll choose (assuming you have more than one possibility). So here's a quick pre-travel checklist.

▸ Athletic shoes

▸ Sweat socks

▸ Jockstraps

▸ Swimsuit and goggles

▸ Shorts or sweatpants

▸ T-shirts or sweatshirts

▸ Gloves and a hat

▸ Sunscreen and sunglasses

▸ Somewhere to stash your hotel key, ID, and cash, if you don't have pockets in your shorts

▸ Jump rope

▸ Athletic shoes (in case you missed them at the top of the list; nothing's dorkier than wearing cap-toe oxfords on a stairclimber)

Pack all this in a plastic bag to save your suits from B.O. You don't want to smell like a high school locker room when you make that crucial sales presentation.

Bonus tip: If it's likely you'll forget to pack any workout gear at all, leave a bag of old workout clothes in your suitcase between trips, or keep a note in there reminding you to pack them.

Avoid air sickness. Today's airplanes have all the charm of a doctor's waiting room, with a fraction of the magazines.

You and your fellow travelers just want to arrive. On time would be nice, but you'll settle for a safe landing. So the airline food is an afterthought. You know it won't be *good* in any sense of the word. It isn't appetizing, it isn't filling, often it's low in protein and, as a final insult, it's high in carbohydrates that you can't possibly burn off when you're crammed in so tight you can't move.

You can do better. When you make your reservations, ask the airline for a special meal. Choices might include vegetarian, seafood, low-calorie, low-fat, or a fruit plate. There's no extra charge and no hassle if you give them at least 6-hours notice, and the special meals are often tastier and fresher than the regular fare. They probably won't be high-protein, but you can take along your own protein bar. You might take a jar of chunky peanut butter and a spoon, but that draws some strange looks. A can of unsalted nuts can also do the trick. (You know there will only be three peanuts in the package the airline provides.) The point is to eat food that makes you less hungry, rather than more.

Walk when you can. If you're not in a rush to make a connection, skip the moving sidewalks and escalators; instead, walk to your gate under your own power. Simply using your muscles and getting your blood pumping can take some of the edge off travel.

Another option, if you have a long layover, is to squeeze in a workout. Many major airports actually have on-site or nearby gyms that you can use for a small fee of anywhere from $7 to $20. See page 182 for a list of gyms near the 25 largest airports in North America.

Once you reach your hotel, get a map of the city and walk or jog around town. And when you go out to eat, pick restaurants you can walk to.

Make your hotel a health club. Hotel gyms are often disappointing. You're lucky if you get a couple of treadmills and a 20-year-old Universal machine crammed into a room that used to be the housekeepers' smoking lounge.

So you may want to go for a day pass at whatever full-service gym is nearby. Sometimes the hotel will have a relationship with a local club and offer complimentary passes. If you belong to a gym chain, of course, you can search for a franchise near your hotel. You may discover it's simpler and cheaper to pay for a day pass somewhere else, but it doesn't hurt to check.

Some guys opt for exercise in their hotel rooms. Most of us can get a pretty

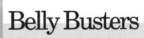

Belly Busters

▶▶ "Fitness and health have ceased to be a chore and now are a welcome part of my life. I never miss an opportunity to exercise; and I take my workout clothes with me on all of my trips, both vacation and business."◀◀

—NICK LEWIS
35, LOST 70 POUNDS

good workout with pushups, lunges, squats, and crunches or situps for the chest, shoulders, triceps, abs, and lower body. If you brought a set of exercise bands, you can hook them around a doorknob and work your back muscles and biceps, too.

Serious road exercisers can bring along a doorway chinup bar to give their backs and arms a good going-over. Advanced guys might also consider plyometric pushups (push up so hard that your hands come off the floor), jump squats, and jump lunges (switch leg positions in midair so you go from a lunge with your right leg forward to a lunge with your left forward, and repeat).

Airport	Where to Exercise	Cost of a Gym Day Pass
Charlotte/Douglas	Gold's Gym, 15-min taxi ride from the airport	$15
Cincinnati/N. Kentucky	Fit Works Fitness and Sports Therapy, 10-min taxi ride	$10
Dallas/Ft. Worth	Irving Fitness, 10-min taxi ride	$10
Denver	Stapleton Fitness Center in the Radisson Hotel, 15-minute free shuttle ride	$10
Detroit Metropolitan	Wayne Racquet & Exercise Club, 15-min taxi ride	$7
George Bush (Houston)	Wyndham Greenspoint, 15-min free shuttle ride	$14
Hartsfield Atlanta	Perimeter Summit Health Club, 25-min taxi ride	$5
Honolulu	Gold's Gym, 10-min taxi ride	$10
JFK (New York City)	Cross Island Sports & Fitness, 10-min taxi ride	$10
LaGuardia (New York City)	LaGuardia Marriott, across the street from the airport	$20
Lambert–St. Louis	St. Louis Workout, 20-min taxi ride	$10
Lester B. Pearson (Toronto)	Curzons Fitness, 5-min taxi ride	$10
Logan (Boston)	Hilton Hotel, 5-min free shuttle ride	$9
Los Angeles	24-Hour Fitness at the Hilton Los Angeles, 5-min taxi ride	$10
McCarran (Las Vegas)	24-Hour Fitness, in the airport terminal	$15
Miami	Miami Int'l Airport Hotel, airport-terminal concourse E	$8
Minneapolis–St. Paul	Appletree Fitness Center at the Holiday Inn Select, 10-min taxi ride	$6
Newark	Hilton Newark Airport, 15-min free shuttle ride	$10
O'Hare (Chicago)	Hilton Chicago O'Hare Airport, in the airport terminal	$10
Orlando	World Gym, 20-min taxi ride	$10
Philadelphia	New Old City Ironworks, 15-min taxi ride	$10
Salt Lake City	The Firm, 15-min taxi ride	$10
San Francisco	Gold's Gym, 20-min taxi ride	$15
Seattle-Tacoma	Powerhouse Gym & Fitness Center, 5-min taxi ride	$15
Sky Harbor (Phoenix)	Phoenix Suns Athletic Club, 10-min taxi ride	$10

We can't mention those exercises without including the fine print: Don't try plyometric moves unless you've been exercising for at least a year, have no nagging injuries or lingering knee problems, and are very comfortable with the normal versions of the exercises—in other words, don't do jump squats unless you're already good at regular squats.

Make it up as you go. When you travel, it's okay to leave your training log at home. You have no way of knowing whether the gym you'll use will have the equipment you need, so you don't have to perform your regular program.

Before you go to the gym, come up with a general idea about what you want to do: which muscles you want to work, whether you want to lift heavy or light, whether you want a real sweatfest or something a little more rejuvenating. Decide on specific exercises and sequences when you walk in the door and see how things are arranged, how crowded the place is, and how you feel at that moment. If you're a few hours removed from a stressful flight, you may need all your workout time to just feel normal again. So the entire workout may be an extended version of your usual warmup—lots of stretches and light sets.

Or you may want to go for the exercise equivalent of comfort food: exercises you like, a favorite old configuration you haven't used in years. Rather than doing what's good for you, you switch to what's fun.

It's not the only way to exercise on the road, but it gives you a reason to look forward to a trip, rather than dread it.

Eat out, but don't cave in. Give yourself one dinner in which you order whatever tempts you. The thought of that one uninhibited feast will make it a lot easier to order good but less tantalizing food the rest of the time.

YOU VERSUS BURNOUT
Burnout is a triumph disguised as a defeat. You think your program has failed you. In reality, it's succeeded so well that you need to move on to something else.

First comes physiological burnout, where your body gets used to a routine and stops making progress. Progress is success, and success is the most important motivational tool you have.

When the success stops, you no longer feel rewarded for your effort, and psychological burnout sets it. Let's face it: Exercise is hard work. If you don't feel that it's rewarding work, why do it? At least those *Family Ties* reruns on Nick at Night give you a few chuckles. And you don't have to launder sweaty clothes after an hour of TV (we hope)

It's possible to go years without hitting either physiological or psychological burnout. You just have to know the warning signs and try like hell to head them off so the rewards of exercise keep coming your way.

Throw yourself a change-up. An entry-level weight-training program has a shelf life of 6 to 8 weeks. The more advanced you become, the quicker the expiration date arrives. So if you start doing the workouts in chapter 11 on July 1, figure that you're going to need to adjust the program sometime around Labor Day.

Problem is, guys like to stick with a program that initially delivered results—no matter how long ago it stopped delivering. The worst-case scenario is that many of the guys who start this program on July 1 will still be doing it on July 1 of next year.

The first sign that a program has stopped working is that you can't increase the weights anymore and end up doing exercises with the same load 2 weeks in a row. If you don't change at that point, you'll find yourself skipping a few repetitions here, maybe a set there. Next thing you know, you'll be coming up with excuses to skip entire workouts.

When you're stuck with the same weights for 2 weeks in a row, change. Here are three ways to freshen up a program.

1. Increase the weights and decrease the reps. You can do this as straight sets or as a pyramid (sets of 12, 8, 6, 4, and 2 repetitions). It's tremendously motivating either way, since you get to work with heavier weights and your body almost immediately responds in both appearance and performance.

2. Of course, you also reach diminishing returns with heavy weights soon enough, so then you can change it up again. One technique that's getting a lot of attention now is changing speeds.

Try lifting lighter weights at slower speeds for a couple of weeks, and see if that produces results. (It probably will . . . for a couple of weeks.) You can also try lifting at faster speeds on some exercises. (Don't try this on any exercise that puts your lower back in jeopardy.)

3. Bodybuilders have known for years about the value of dividing up your muscle groups so you work different muscles on different days. For 6 months, try working different muscles on different days, aiming to hit everything once a week. (This is called a split routine.) For the next 6 months, work all muscles each time you're in the gym. Don't do the same exercises more than one workout per week. The latter technique was used in Craig Ballantyne's workouts in chapter 11, while the former system is shown in workouts designed by Michael Mejia in the book *The Testosterone Advantage Plan*.

When you've hit the wall using one of these techniques, it's a good bet you can start making progress again by switching to another. Whichever workout system you haven't used recently is the one that will most likely work best for you now.

Find some new scenery. Endurance-oriented exercisers get into ruts, too. Same route, same time of day, same distance, same speed. So the first path out of your rut is a change in one of those variables. Shorter treks through hillier terrain turn a steady-effort workout into more of an interval routine.

Be your own toughest competition. Researchers have found that athletes who compete against themselves and focus their efforts on getting better are more likely to maintain interest and work harder. For example, if you enjoy cycling for fitness, try training for a mountain-bike race. The added challenge of improving your bike-handling skills and trying to top your fastest ride times may be very motivating for you.

If you lift weights, you probably won't enter a competition, but that doesn't mean you can't set out to increase your maximum bench press, deadlift, or squat.

Sometimes, just be. In general, performance goals are great motivational tools. The more you try to accomplish, the more you will accomplish. However, when a tightly regimented routine starts to feel stale, it helps to back off on the goals and simply enjoy the feeling of exercise again. In the weight room, you can go for a cheap pump: Do a bunch of bodybuilder exercises, and relish the sensation of your muscles engorging with blood. On the road, you can relax and take in the scenery.

Play sports. Many guys find that there's something about sports that's more deeply satisfying than any other type of physical activity. Most exercise is repetitive and two-dimensional—back and forth, up and down. There aren't many variables. But in games such as basketball, soccer, tennis, hockey, or football, you never repeat the same play twice. You may try, but the fact that you're playing against somebody who reacts differently each time means every sequence plays out a little differently.

Belly Busters

▶▶"I am constantly learning new exercises to keep myself from getting bored and to work slightly different muscle groups."◀◀

—JONATHAN COLEMAN
25, LOST 39 POUNDS

And even in a solo sport like golf, you never attempt the same exact shot twice.

The result is a full engagement of mind and body. Hour-long games seem to end a minute after they start. You burn hundreds of calories without any conscious effort. You're just playing.

Playing sports isn't a normal part of adult life for many of us—few businesses are set up to accommodate lunchtime pickup games or even after-work leagues. And a lot of us have endured negative athletic experiences dating back to our pre-jockstrap days. We were the last guys picked in dodge ball, were relegated to two innings in right field in Little League, and were generally knocked around and otherwise humiliated by bigger, stronger, more naturally athletic kids.

Nevertheless, if you get out there with buddies, sports can be transforming. When the game is over, the feeling of satisfaction and replenishment is deeper than from any other type of activity. That feeling is what really matters. No matter how you get it, you want to bask in the thought that what you did was fun, significant, and replicable. That's what can keep you exercising for a lifetime.

A Formerly Round All-Around Athlete

LIFE IN THE FAT LANE

After graduation, high school jock Steve Hanzir remembers, he took up three unhealthy extracurricular activities: beer, wings, and the recliner. "I didn't have football or wrestling practice, and the only running I was doing was to the refrigerator," he admits. Though his job at a paper mill was physical, working the graveyard shift had him dead on his feet. After a long night unloading trucks, he'd drag himself home at 7:00 A.M., eat, and then fall into bed.

Before long, the former athlete weighed more than 300 pounds. "The only shape I was in was round," he says.

THE TURNING POINT

In December of 2000, Hanzir's weight caught up with him during a hunting trip, when the deer and his buddies all outran him. "I'm going through 6 inches of snow, breaking through the ice, and going down through another foot of snow. . . . They were going like rabbits across the top of the ridge. . . . I was keeping up with them for a little while. Then I just watched them get farther and farther ahead. I couldn't breathe. . . . I just thought for sure I was going to die. And the more I thought about it, the madder I got at myself."

That anger got Hanzir off the mountain and even helped him bag an eight-point buck. But it wasn't quite enough to motivate him to get back in shape.

The final incentive turned up a few days later, when he saw a photo of himself and his son putting up the Christmas tree. "That made me decide that it was either get off my ass and start taking care of myself or probably miss my kids growing up."

He headed to the weight room the next day.

THE PLAN OF ATTACK

Thanks to his years on the gridiron and the wrestling mat, Hanzir knew what he had to do to get back to his fighting weight. Almost every day, he hit the weights for 20 to 30 minutes, doing two or three exercises for each muscle group and two or three sets of each exercise. "That way, I'm still working enough where it's cutting up and it looks good, but I'm not bulking up either." He worked a different

Name: Steve Hanzir
Occupation: Laborer and assistant junior high football coach
Residence: Tyrone, Pennsylvania
Date of Birth: December 1971
Height: 5 foot 10

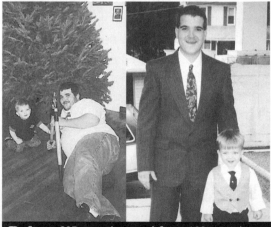

Before: 305 pounds   **After:** 198 pounds

muscle group each day: arms and chest one day; shoulders, back, and lats the next; and legs the day after that.

He also did 10 to 15 minutes' worth of ab work and, though he hated it, started running. "It was like a fast walk or slow jog—I called it a wog."

His wrestling experience helped him revamp his diet as well. "When I wrestled and I had to cut weight, I knew the proper way to do it. We had a real good coach. He didn't push us too hard, but he educated us as far as the right way to do things—what you should and shouldn't eat, while not starving yourself and not dehydrating."

Hanzir ate more fruits and vegetables, plus high-protein, low-fat, and low-sugar choices such as cereal, tuna, and fat-free bologna and hot dogs. "The fat-free stuff nowadays tastes a whole lot better than what that crap used to taste like," he says. Hanzir stopped eating before bed, making sure his last meal of the day was 4 to 5 hours before he turned in.

His efforts gave him a sporting chance to get back to the athletic shape he'd once had: Within 6 months, he had lost more than 70 pounds.

"It was easy at that point. I just broke all the old, bad habits and got into the good ones. I was seeing results at that point, and there was no way I was going back to what I was doing before."

LIFE IN THE FIT LANE

A year after that fateful day on the mountain, Hanzir had reduced his pants size from a "tight, tight" 42 to a 34. "I was wearing 36s my senior year, when I graduated. So I'm in better shape than I've ever been in my life."

Hanzir feels so good that he's even sought new running challenges, despite his initial dislike for the sport. "I ran a 5-K race over the summer, just to be able to say I did it," he says. He not only did it but also came in fifth or sixth in his age group. Even better, he beat an old high school wrestling rival who had also run cross-country. "I didn't see him at the start, but I passed him during the race. So I was sitting at the finish line waiting for him, just to let him know it. He was one of the lightweights who was always messing with the heavier guys."

Hanzir's competitors aren't the only guys who've been surprised by his renewed athleticism. As an assistant junior high football coach, he runs with the team. In the past, it was easy for the players to keep up with him. Not anymore, as Hanzir discovered when a young lineman expressed his disappointment with his leaner, fitter coach. "He said, 'I liked you better when you were fat. You understood the plight of a fat man.'"

Hanzir says he hadn't even noticed that he was challenging his team to work harder. But the kid did have a point: Hanzir understands the plight of the fat man well enough to know he doesn't ever want to experience it again.

HIS TIPS

GO WILD. "I eat a lot of game and venison because there's less fat in that meat than there is in other stuff."

PACE YOURSELF. "Every other week or so, if I felt like wings and a beer, I'd have wings and a beer. But I wouldn't go buy a case and have it gone by the end of the weekend. I limited myself."

Index

Underscored page reference indicate boxed text. **Boldface** references indicate photographs.

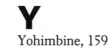